MW01413289

RESTORATIVE HEALING BEGINS WITH REST

Overcoming Breathing difficulties
and PTSD after 9/11 exposure

ORAL PATRICK,
DEBORAH PATRICK

Copyright © 2022 Oral Patrick, Deborah Patrick.

All rights reserved. No part of this book may be used or reproduced by any means, graphic, electronic, or mechanical, including photocopying, recording, taping or by any information storage retrieval system without the written permission of the author except in the case of brief quotations embodied in critical articles and reviews.

Consult your doctor and do your own research before attempting any of the practices in this book. The techniques provided are ones he has attempted for his personal healing.

Balboa Press books may be ordered through booksellers or by contacting:

Balboa Press
A Division of Hay House
1663 Liberty Drive
Bloomington, IN 47403
www.balboapress.com
844-682-1282

Because of the dynamic nature of the Internet, any web addresses or links contained in this book may have changed since publication and may no longer be valid. The views expressed in this work are solely those of the author and do not necessarily reflect the views of the publisher, and the publisher hereby disclaims any responsibility for them.

The author of this book does not dispense medical advice or prescribe the use of any technique as a form of treatment for physical, emotional, or medical problems without the advice of a physician, either directly or indirectly. The intent of the author is only to offer information of a general nature to help you in your quest for emotional and spiritual well-being. In the event you use any of the information in this book for yourself, which is your constitutional right, the author and the publisher assume no responsibility for your actions.

Any people depicted in stock imagery provided by Getty Images are models, and such images are being used for illustrative purposes only.
Certain stock imagery © Getty Images.

Print information available on the last page.

ISBN: 979-8-7652-2659-9 (sc)
ISBN: 979-8-7652-2658-2 (hc)
ISBN: 979-8-7652-2669-8 (e)

Library of Congress Control Number: 2022910202

Balboa Press rev. date: 06/01/2022

CONTENTS

Preface vii
Introduction xv

1. Body 1
    1.1 Toxicity and Elimination 2
    1.2 Sleep: The Rhythm of Life 4
    1.3 Life and Death Begins in the Gut 8
    1.4 Life in Motion 13
    1.5 Water-Based Feasting 18
    1.6 Breathing in the Life Force 30

2. Mind 33
    2.1 Emotionally Balanced 34
    2.2 Musication: Music as Medicine 40
    2.3 The Placebo: Belief Kills and Belief Cures 43
    2.4 Meditation: Quiet the Mind 47
    2.5 What Frequency Are You On? 50
    2.6 As a Person Thinks 55

3. Spirit 61
    3.1 In-spirit-ation or Inspiration 61
    3.2 Authenticity 64
    3.3 Faith Conquers Fear 68
    3.4 Vision Transcends the Past 75
    3.5 Ascendence 80
    3.6 The Dance of Bliss 85

PREFACE

9/11 Conqueror, not Survivor

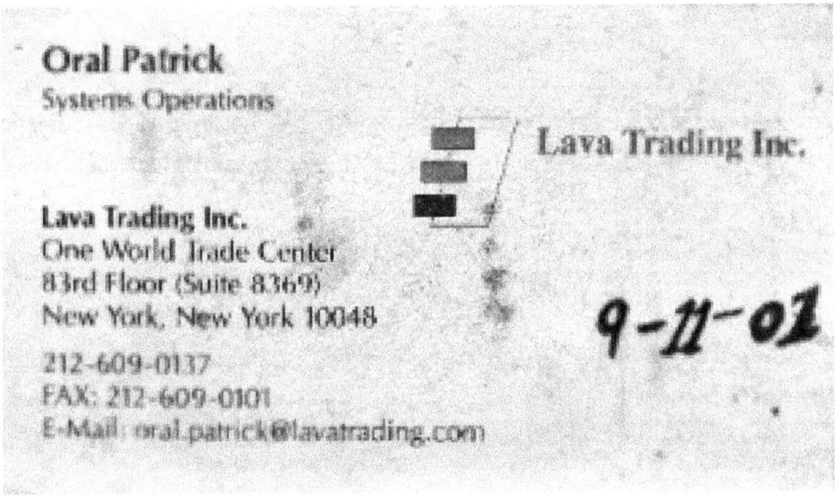

Figure 1. Business Card

It's September 10, 2001, and I'd just been terminated from my job as a computer technologist. I previously worked on the eighty-third floor of the World Trade Center in lower Manhattan. I had no idea that the next day, planes would shatter the buildings and kill many of the occupants on my floor. This resulted in my life shattering and soon spinning out of control. The chaos of 9/11 was a perfect metaphor for my life.

Here's the full story. On the morning of September 10, my manager called me into the conference room shortly after 9 a.m., as soon as he entered the office. He said the company was in the process of laying off, and I was the first one to go. He asked me to sign my resignation letter. He told security to escort me to my desk to collect my personal belongings. I have never been fired before. All kinds of thoughts were going through my head: *Why me? What did I do wrong? What am I going to do now? How will I pay my bills?*

However, I packed my stuff and mustered the courage to salute the team goodbye as I left the office. I called my brother, and we went to a favorite restaurant and celebrated what I hoped would be a new beginning.

The next morning, in what started out as a beautiful fall day with a light breeze, the sun had just peeked out. I was on my way back into the city to put in some job applications and to network. Shortly after 8 a.m., as I was driving on the NJ Turnpike, I glanced toward the landmark WTC Twin Towers in the distance, thinking how I could be at work there right now had I not gotten fired the day before.

Then, as I looked again, I saw a strange smoke emanating from the towers. *That is rather strange,* I thought. So I turned to a local news radio station to get an update. The reporters initially thought a small plane may have gone off course and accidentally hit one of the towers. But later, they announced that something more sinister seemed to be at work.

Traffic was soon diverted and eventually came to a standstill as all tunnels and bridges to the downtown were closed. So I parked, went to a nearby deli restaurant, and watched the live news being shown on the deli's TV, the towers in the distance.

All the TV networks were broadcasting live from the scene, showing the pandemonium: whaling sirens, emergency lights flashing, circling news choppers, and thick dust in the air as first responders intervened. I was shocked to see people on fire jumping from several stories above ground as black and red roaring flames licked the upper portion of both towers. I imagined my former coworkers trying to find a way to escape and asking themselves who caused this as they were being burned to death. And I wondered what would have happened to me if I were in the building. Maybe some were thinking to call their families and friends and tell them goodbye. We would later learn that some did so.

Just after 9 a.m., as the waiter handed me my pancakes and eggs, I saw the first tower come down before my eyes, like a house of cards. Many restaurant patrons, who were watching also, screamed in utter disbelief. I fell on my knees in a fetal position. Then I put my hands on my head for a long time, trying to process what I just saw. I had no frame of reference for what I had just seen.

Then shortly after that, the second tower fell. I spent several stunned hours in the deli before I went back uptown and headed home that afternoon.

In the ensuing days and weeks, I went back to the area around ground zero to see if I could assist with search and rescue efforts for friends and coworkers who could still be trapped under rubble. The scents of burning flesh and plastic were traumatizing. The sight of tons of debris from the fallen buildings was unbelievable, and sounds of sirens were everywhere. As a result, I got chronically ill from the pollutants in the air and the emotional stress of daily life. Unfortunately, several thousand of the 9/11 victims and hero rescuers succumbed to the toxins that caused respiratory, skin, and digestive cancers and other health issues. God bless our heroes!

At this point, not only was I physically and mentally hurting and stressed out, but I was overleveraged in many other areas of my life. Having lost my job and with the economy staggering from the 9/11 attacks and the stock market closed for the first time in decades before taking a record plunge, I was financially depleted. My late-model car was repossessed, and I was at the point of foreclosure on and eviction from my condo.

Additionally, I was emotionally stressed out because my lifelong relationship was conflicted and now on the rocks. I moved out of town and was separated from my spiritual community of friends and family. It was very humbling, even humiliating. In short, I had hit a new rock bottom.

My life had become like a long stormy night that would not end. I continued to experience debilitating symptoms of skin rashes and respiratory congestion. I was also slightly overweight and prediabetic. And I experienced many subclinical conditions, like gut microbiome disruption, that doctors were not able to measure and assess easily and were contributing to my constant fatigue.

Having made little or no progress with the regular medical methods, I poured myself into the world of natural healing and started an in-depth study of wellness and how to overcome chronic illness. I spent a tremendous amount of time in research, including seeking experts in various areas of health, with the goal of healing myself. As a result, I have become very knowledgeable about this subject as a medical journalist.

After consulting with natural health practitioners, I learned that almost any device will work again if you unplug it for a while and then reboot it—even our bodies. I was thinking about the caterpillar who crawls under a leaf and sits in a dark quiet place for a few days with no external interference. It gets rested and rebooted. It cocoons and is transformed into a butterfly with no external input, just the software of divine intelligence transforming the hardware. So I decided to put rest to the test.

It was now more than a full year since 9/11. I realized that conventional methods were not relieving my symptoms. Instead, they worsened. I was still experiencing severe respiratory congestion, which made breathing difficult. There was skin discoloration on different parts of my body, including my arms and face. But then things changed during one remarkable week. I had been totally exhausted and stayed in bed for more than a week with little or no food or activity; I was unable to do much. Then I started to hope against all odds and came to a place of gratitude for wholeness and life. I will never forget the day I started to notice the significant changes after one week of resting my body, mind, and spirit.

I woke up thinking this would be yet another day spent in bed. Instead, I found that my mood, sight, hearing, appearance, and mental clarity were transformed. I experienced a spiritual and emotional reboot and restoration! I threw off the blanket, jumped out of bed, and ran to the window to absorb the beautiful sunshine coming up from behind the mountain in the distance. I took a deep breath of the spring air and exhaled with a new passion for life. I threw my hands up in the air and spontaneously began to say, "Thank you," for a new life and a new body. I felt like someone who had been thrown a lifeline just before going under.

As I walked around my room, I felt elated. My depressed mood was lifted, a sense of emotional well-being overwhelmed me, and I felt like dancing and singing! My body felt so light and buoyant that I wanted to jump. And I did in fact jump up and was able to spring much higher than I have ever recalled. I realized that my joints, which were previously arthritic, were pain-free and more flexible once I moved around.

As I continued to look out at the lush green vegetation, I saw shades and hues of light that was out of this world and that I was not able to perceive before. The fog was lifted, and the world took on a glow and seemed brighter.

A familiar song was playing on my music device. I was able to hear harmonies and sound of decibels that I was not able to hear before.

The discolored patches on my hand were significantly reduced and went away a few days later. Even my hair became noticeably thicker. My breathing was much less forced as stuffiness and bleeding became negligible. I was awed and filled with amazement!

When I started to eat breakfast, I noticed that the food tasted so delicious. My tastebuds seemed to have been revitalized.

I noticed that I was able to solve problems and see patterns much faster. The following week, I was working on a manual-writing project. I had been unable to make much progress over the past few months because of brain fog and lack of mental clarity. However, as I sat at my desk that morning, I had so much mental clarity and acuity that I grabbed my notebook and was pretty much able to write the entire manual in under an hour.

A month later, I was at a gathering with some friends I had not seen in a few weeks. One of them started looking at me rather questioningly, and his jaw dropped! Then he asked me, "You look so different! How did you lose the excess weight? Why do you look so amazingly different?"

I told him about the power of spiritual, emotional, and physical rest and how I used it to restore myself. He tried some of my suggestions a few weeks later and got amazing results. So he asked me to document it so it can be shared with a wider audience.

Later in the summer, I was reunited with my wife and family. Besides being incredibly beautiful, she is witty, playful, provocative, and very caring. And from the day I met her, I knew that she always has my back. When you are on a team, one of the persons who always gets picked first is the most helpful person. That is the person who has your back. Relationships are strengthened not only by the good times but also by the bad times we endure and survive. As a couple, we do not hide our heads in the sand and pretend that problems don't exist or that each other is perfect. Instead, we lovingly confront and challenge each other to be our best selves. I am not suggesting that this may not sometimes result in verbal fights or conflicts of opinions, but it allows us to understand each other more and appreciate our differences.

Now that I have been healed, my goal is to serve my community by sharing the life lessons I have garnered. My entrepreneurial ventures were born out of a desire to serve and teach my friends and family so that they don't have to make the same mistakes as I did. My goal is service, not fame and fortune.

Two years later, I started a computer cybersecurity company that provides consultations for Fortune 50 companies. Additionally, due to post-9/11 high demand for living space outside the city, I established a real estate investment company to address that need. Eventually, I founded Word Of Wisdom (WOW), a nonprofit organization dedicated to the healing and self-restoration of the body, mind, and spirit, where I, as a life coach, present and interactively share words of wisdom that I have learned from the great minds of the world on a regular basis in person and via social media. I know that adversity does not have to be the final chapter in our book because we can overcome adversity and be restored to an even greater life. Rest has transformed my life in ways that I had only dreamed of.

Recently, the money that the government allocated for the 9/11 victims ran out. Several of the affected first responders succumbed to lung cancer because of inhaling toxic smoke during the cleanup of ground zero. Luckily, while many of my counterparts who lived and worked in and around the area of attack, succumbed to various chronic conditions, I was able to rest and reboot by applying some amazingly effective techniques. And now, my health has been fully restored. I detail some of these techniques in the following pages.

I would like to thank my family and friends for their contribution to this book.

Here are few questions about your level of restfulness. For each question, you can rate yourself on a scale of 1 to 10.

> Do you fall asleep quickly after going to bed?
> Do you get at least seven to eight hours of sleep per night?
> Do you wake up feeling revived and refreshed?
> Is your diet based largely on water-based foods?
> Are you free from chronic pain in all areas of your body?
> Do you feel emotionally unstable and angry for most of the day?
> Do you take time to give the body exercise and movement?
> How flexible are the joints in your body?
> How exhausted are you at the end of a typical work day?
> Do you spend time on a daily or weekly basis to meditate and connect?

If you score below 50 or answered no to any of these questions, this book is definitely for you.

If you scored between 50 and 80, this book can be of value to you.

If you scored 80 to 100, then you are doing great, but this book still has something to offer you.

If you scored over 100, then you may be able to teach us something.

When you are finished reading this book, you will gain the following benefits:

- Learn to live longer and healthier.
- Understand the inexpensive way to overcome chronic illnesses.
- Have better sleep.
- Have more peace of mind and mental clarity.
- Connect with super-consciousness.
- Enjoy deeper relationships with loved ones.
- Feel more rested and alive.
- Access higher states of spiritual awareness for guidance.

Thanks to all my friends and family who help to make this book a success. This book is dedicated to my supportive wife, Angella, and my children Elizabeth, Prince, Esther, and Deborah

INTRODUCTION

> The best of all medicines are resting and fasting.
>
> —Benjamin Franklin

A sick and tired billionaire on his deathbed, in his early sixties, spoke about the book about *Rest* that he realized he had not yet read and wished he had. Of all the books that he had read on business, technology, money, leadership, travel, fine lifestyle, history, and so on, this was the book that eluded him, and he regretted it the most. This was one of the most important books that he thought he should have read.

As I talk to friends and associates daily, I sometimes get a sense of their disillusionment and disenchantment regarding their own health and well-being. Many times, people don't know the root cause of their sicknesses even after many clinical diagnostics. And even if the doctor can name it, he or she may not have a cure. Therefore, I want them to understand that the solution to wellness has more to do with rest, homeostasis, than with any external concoction we can take. We can create wellness when we remove the mental, emotional, and physiological toxins that result in disease. The science is truly clear on this. And I, along with many others, have proven this time and time again in our experiences. This very simple, straightforward, and inexpensive, but very effective method hides in plain sight in a time when we are programmed to believe we need to do something like take a drug or have an operation for everything that ails us. In medical school, it is taught that there is a, "pill for every ill," and a, "shot for every sickness." However, our natural innate immune systems can assist in recovery and disease prevention when it is strengthened through rest.

The pandemic caused by the COVID-19 virus exacerbated the inherent flaws in our health and health systems. A large percentage of the patients admitted with COVID-19 had some sort of underlying chronic illness condition. I was able to share some information with a few people infected by this virus, and it has been very helpful in their recoveries. Friends who I have previously shared it with were able to avoid infection in conjunction with all the best practices and precautions needed to prevent infection.

What Is Real Restorative Rest?

Restorative rest incorporates a mind-body-spirit solution, not just the body, based on my research and experiments. Rest is not merely closing your eyes and falling asleep. Yes, physical rest involves this and much more. But notice that even sleep involves taking the body away from any kind of noise, distraction, or activity. So a more comprehensive perspective of rest is to place, not only the body, but also the mind and spirit in a state of inactivity and tranquility. Whenever this occurs, all aspects of our beings are able to properly repair themselves and restore our bodies to proper functioning and health almost magically.

All the systems of the body naturally move toward balance, homeostasis, and health when given a chance. Newton's first law of motion implies that a body remains in a state of rest unless acted upon by external forces. And when the external disturbance is removed, it reverts to equilibrium. Like a pendulum when the external force is removed, it comes to a standstill after a time. The longer the rest and inactivity, the deeper and more complete the healing. There is a place for activity, but it must be balanced by a proper cycle of rest. The body experiences its own cycle of rest and activity called the circadian rhythm, which we will discuss at length in a later chapter. It has been proven that animals in hibernation automatically experience an increase in healing hormones and stem cells that restore their body systems.

Besides sleep, resting the body involves resting the digestive system, which means that we need to periodically stay away from any food that activates the digestive process. Even when we are asleep, our digestive systems may sometimes still be at work, depending on the time we eat. Prolonged abstinence from food allows the body's energy to directly repair the brain and the body in general. When our brains are functioning optimally, we have a sense of euphoria and emotional and spiritual bliss.

Emotional disturbances can effectively throw the body out of balance just as easily as chemical imbalances and create aberrations. Our world is experiencing an astonishing amount of chronic degenerative diseases. Illnesses like heart disease, obesity, diabetes, cancer, and dementia are increasing. Almost everyone has had a bout with at least one of these conditions or know people who have. Most people just assume these are only normal signs of aging, and the conventional medical system has no solution when it comes to preventing or easily recovering from these conditions.

Our bodies were created with incredible innate abilities to heal themselves. Our lifestyle and habits disrupt this innate healing process as we overload our bodies with metabolic and other toxins. Many over-the-counter products contain ingredients that are damaging to one's health. These ingredients may not be on the label, and labels may not even state that they are damaging to our bodies.

In this time of fear and uncertainty, there lies an incredible opportunity to heal on physical, emotional, and spiritual levels. In this book, you will discover the different techniques of rest and how to apply them in very specific ways to activate the body's self-healing mechanisms and balance the systems of the body.

People all over the world are looking for real, permanent answers to health issues such as chronic pain, dementia, diabetes, anxiety, cancer, periodontal disease, and skin problems. And the great thing about these rest techniques is that they do not require any expensive medical processes or concoctions, and they are substantiated by medical science.

1

BODY

ALL THE FOLKS WHO WERE around the fallen towers for several days and weeks had inhaled toxic chemicals. Not only were their respiratory systems overwhelmed, the toxins lodged all over their bodies, affecting other organs, such as the skin, eyes, liver, and kidneys. Medication was not as effective for me because my body was so overwhelmed. My body only had enough energy to deal with regular digestion and elimination of the food that I was putting into it. But once I rested my digestive system by reducing and eliminating my food intake, all my life force went into clearing up these organs.

One of the most common things that causes unrest, distress, disease, and dis-ease to the human body is toxic food. Foods that are difficult or impossible for the digestive system to assimilate become or produce toxic residue that throws off the body's biochemical balance. This residue can later become a substrate that attracts microorganisms that ingest these toxins and produce more toxins as the product of their excretions. However, the body has an innate ability to heal itself, and it is constantly attempting to heal itself and return to a place of balance, homeostasis, and rest. If it is given the chance, and if it is not overwhelmed, it can effectively eliminate toxins. So when we reduce or eliminate the input of food, the body uses its life force to cleanse itself. But if we constantly introduce things into our bodies, this energy goes first into digestion before it starts the elimination process. Depending on how fast we introduce food to our bodies, it may never get to truly eliminate the toxins, so they begin to pile up. It is like our homes; we need to balance our efforts between bringing in new stuff and cleaning up and taking out the garbage we generate. If we bring in a lot of stuff—even good stuff—faster than we take out garbage, our houses will become messy and places of unease because there will be no time or energy left over to clean.

A person may think that the best way to health is to introduce a new concoction. But it is impossible for the body to properly use this new stuff if it is still in the process of moving out the garbage from the previous cycle. Even though it may seem counterintuitive, the best way to achieve clarity and balance is to allow the body to clear out the old before we bring in the new.

1.1 Toxicity and Elimination

> This is the rest where you may cause the weary to rest; and this is the refreshing.
>
> —Isiah

Toxicity is ubiquitous in today's environment. Our internal and external environments create feeding and breeding grounds for organisms like bacteria and viruses and other pathogens. The liver deals with toxins, and when it is overloaded, these toxins are deposited on other organs, causing skin issues, joint stiffness, ear problems, dental issues, and shadows in the eyes. When these toxins are eliminated, the body can get back to its state of rest and homeostasis, which allows it to heal itself.

Every machine comes with a manual that tells us how to operate it. For instance, you should not put oil in the gasoline tank of the car. And you should not put excessive air in a tire or else it will not function properly. In fact, it will break the car. Likewise, there are things that we should not put into or on our bodies because they will cause them to malfunction. Even the things that are good for our bodies should be used in moderation, not excessively. If something placed into the body causes it to malfunction, you should eliminate it, and allow the body enough rest so that the healing process can do a complete job.

For example, many degenerative diseases, such as high blood pressure and diabetes, that are caused or exacerbated by excessive salt and sugar can be reversed or mitigated by reducing salt and sugar intake. Diabetes, which correlates to or worsens Alzheimer's, can be minimized with reduced sugar intake. One of my clients mentioned to me that he had high blood pressure. He went to a doctor and was given a prescription that helped with the pressure. After a few months, he experienced elevated blood pressure again. He went back to the doctor and was given a stronger prescription. So I asked him about his salt intake. After reducing his salt and saturated fat intake, like butter, he started to feel better, and his blood pressure went down. He went back to the doctor, and the doctor took him off the blood pressure medication.

After I was exposed to the toxins of the 9/11 WTC bombings, my condition deteriorated even though I was taking prescription medication. A big part of my recovery involved colonic hydration enemas, which my neuropathic doctor introduced me to, combined with other detoxification herbs that can accelerate the elimination of toxins from the body, allowing it to rapidly return to homeostasis.

Blue Zones

Many of us get burned out and expire prematurely because we don't take time to turn off our engines and let them cool down for service before we fire them up again. We overrun our engines and burn ourselves out. The life expectancy of the average American is about seventy-eight years. The blue zones represent pockets of people in various parts of the world who, on average, live beyond one hundred years. Studies have shown that life expectancy is determined by environmental factors more than genetic factors. People in these blue zones have diets that are largely plant-based, and they are typically nonsmokers, which reduces the amount of toxic intake. They also live a relaxed lifestyle and use as much natural stuff as possible.

1.2 Sleep: The Rhythm of Life

> Each night, when I go to sleep, I die. And the next morning, when I wake up, I am reborn.
>
> —Mahatma Gandhi

Our bodies follow a natural pattern called the circadian rhythm, which govern our sleep and awake cycles. We produce certain chemicals based on the body's reaction to visible light. When light hits the eye, the brain produces serotonin. When light is removed, the pineal gland in the center of the brain is energized to produce melatonin, which causes the body to sleep. Melatonin can be further energized and converted into other chemicals that can be found in hibernating animals not using their energy for moving, procreating, or eating. These chemicals are powerful antiaging, hallucinogenic, photoluminescent chemicals.

For the weeks leading up to 9/11, I was waking up extra early, working long hours, and getting little or no rest in order to take care of my family. I wore my constant exhaustion as a badge of honor for diligence. My parents, who were immigrants, instilled hard work ethics in us by example.

I was experiencing chronic fatigue, which was further compounded by the events surrounding 9/11. Many symptoms of chronic burnout are subclinical. That is, they may not show up on standard clinical diagnostic tests such as X-rays and CAT scans. For instance, I became cranky, and I found it difficult to climb a few steps. I eventually got so ill that I did not have a choice but to lie in bed, and I developed a new appreciation for rest and rediscovered the vitality of sleep. Now I have created a routine that flows with my natural circadian rhythms. Sleep boosts our moods and our immunities.

Circadian Cycles

Everything in nature has a cycle that makes it effective. For many centuries, before the industrial revolution, our ancestors' activities were centered around the sun's cycles, and this has been cemented in our genes. We have lived on an earth that, for millions of years, has had alternating periods of light and darkness every twenty-four hours. Like the animals, our sleeping, feeding, and resting times were based on the light provided by the sun. Notice that you might get jet lag whenever you go to another part of the world with a different time zone. This is because our bodies need a few days to adjust to the new rhythm.

Jeffrey C. Hall, Michael Rosbash, and Michael W. Young were the joint winners of the 2017 Nobel Prize in physiology or medicine. The won for their discoveries about the internal clocks and biological rhythms that govern human life. The following is from the Nobel Assembly at Karolinska Institute, which makes the announcement every year, https://www.nobelprize.org/prizes/medicine/2017/prize-announcement/ press release.

> With exquisite precision, our inner clock adapts our physiology to the dramatically different phases of the day. The clock regulates critical functions such as behavior, hormone levels, sleep, body temperature and metabolism.

This clock is in every cell of our bodies, and a master clock located in the retinal receptors connected to the pineal gland. This means that we must get light in the morning to activate this clock to trigger these processes, and we need darkness at night to tell the body to shut down the system and begin repair. This clock coordinates critical body functions, including heart rate, breathing, and vision.

Additional research shows that when we eat our heaviest meal during the time when the sun is at or near its peak—that is, between 11:00 a.m. and 2:00 p.m.—we get the best results as our digestive juices are at optimal levels. Exposure to blue light from florescent lights and electronic devices late in the night throws the rhythm off. We need downtime for the body to do its repair work, or we break the clock and down-regulate our genes. This clock in the cells tells the body to shut down and stop digestion and begin cleanup and repair.

In the modern world, with so many distractions, we need to systematically create some routine to keep our bodies working optimally. These are just suggestions based on what works for me and many others. There is some flexibility in applying these suggestions to account for the unexpected emergencies or fun times without experiencing guilt trips. If we lack sleep for a few hours each day, our bodies will go into a diseased state.

- Create a daily routine with a fixed time to go to bed and wake up.
- Don't eat after dark; try to eat your heaviest meal when the sun is highest in the sky.
- Reduce exposure to blue light and EM signals at least two hours before bedtime.
- Aim to go to bed close to 10 p.m. and get about eight hours of sleep.
- Don't think about past problems or future issues.
- Take deep breaths, each lasting three to six seconds per cycle.
- Gently rest your mind and imagine your breath going through your body.
- Lie on your back in a relaxed state, with your hands over your stomach or by your side. Lying on your side or stomach will also work.
- Have a comfortable mattress on the harder side not too soft to distort the spine.
- Wear loose clothes and nothing that will restrict blood circulation.
- Use a white noise generator to block distracting sounds.
- Lavender aroma therapy mask to block light
- Make sure the room is the right temperature; cooler is better than warme
- Melatonin tablets may help as a last resort.

Restful Sleep

Are you dreaming of falling asleep as soon as your head hits the pillow? "The well-rested person does not fall asleep immediately," said Rebecca Robbins, an instructor in the division of sleep medicine for Harvard Medical School and coauthor of the book *Sleep for Success!* Normally, a person who gets enough rest each night will slowly drift off to sleep. This can be compared to a person who is well fed and will slowly eat her food, but if she is starving, then she will devour the food very rapidly.

While an occasional afternoon nap is OK, we should try and avoid napping too close to bedtime. Restful sleep is not possible if you wake up often in the night for extended periods, which will prevent you from entering rapid eye movement (REM), or deep delta sleep, where we experience dreams. During this sleep time, your brain rids itself of toxins, and you experience rejuvenation.

If we lack sleep, for instance if you get only four to six hours of sleep per night for just a week, your blood will become so messed up that you could be classified as diabetic. Today, there are many sleep disorders—such as sleep apnea, narcolepsy, and insomnia—which the suggestions above can help to reduce or eliminate since restful sleep allows the brain and body to be repaired.

When we lack sleep, the brain is forced to do something to activate rest. That is why we nod off briefly, as part of our brain goes to sleep. When we lack sleep, one's ability to perform is impaired. Adenosine builds up when we don't sleep, but when we sleep, it is reduced. Caffeine can inhibit adenosine receptors, temporarily creating the illusion of wakefulness.

REM: Sleep on It

When we sleep a short time after learning something, we can later recall what we learned more readily. The best way to illustrate this is using a filing cabinet analogy. When we receive new information, it goes in short-term memory, which is like a limited-capacity inbox. When we sleep, this new information gets sorted out based on various attributes. It is then moved from short-term memory to long term. While short-term memory has limited capacity to hold memories, the long-term memory holds more, so we remember more—*if* we sort stuff out before they spill over and out of short-term memory and are lost. We think better about those who wronged us, and we see different sides to difficult problems after even a brief rest. Melatonin is created in the body when we are about to sleep, and when light hits the eyes, melatonin is converted to serotonin, which causes us to wake up.

Dreams serves an important role in our lives. It is believed that dreams play out extremely emotional positive or negative situations we see and think about as a way of simulating what could happen and how to respond to these situations in real life. When we enter deep sleep, the brain exhibits alpha waves that are characterized by a low frequency and high amplitude. On average, we experience REM sleep every ninety minutes. During REM, the brain flushes out cellular wastes to restore the body to normal function. If you do not get proper rest to experience REM, you may experience disturbing dreams with weird images and sounds that seem very real. This stems from distorted virtual reality signals in the brain.

1.3 Life and Death Begins in the Gut

> Diet is seen as the most powerful way to change your gut microbiome, since each bacterial species feeds on specific foods.
>
> —Deepak Chopra

At conception, one of the first parts of the body that is formed is the gut, otherwise known as the ectoderm, which is the point of attachment of the fetus to the womb. Then the entire body grows from this gut. All disease starts in the gut; all healing starts in the gut. Eighty percent of one's immune system resides in the gut in the form of flora. Therefore, if you boost your gut health by cleansing, which rests the gut, you can be very resistant to environmental toxins, COVID-19, or many other infections for that matter.

In the months prior to 9/11, I was eating lots of fast food such as french fries and pizza, which is not the best definition of healthy eating since they mainly consist of highly processed foods high in carbohydrates and sugar.

Digestion Begins in the Mind

As we prepare food and extend gratitude for our food, we start to salivate and produce the digestive juices to assimilate the food.

Many times, I have gone to a doctor and received a vague diagnosis and given drugs only to still have the condition. The gut, especially the large intestine, consists of millions of microbes, known as the gut flora, that helps to keep the immune system intact. When we ingest foods that are high in pesticides and sodium, it upsets this delicate balance and destroys the gut flora population. Consuming more natural foods allows the gut to rest so this flora can be replenished and regrown. In the United States, yearly deaths from non-communicable diseases like obesity and hypetension which are related to lifestyle, is close to the number of deaths caused by the WTC and Pentagon plane crashes on 9/11. A large percentage of the immune system is in the gut in the form of several pounds of microbiome that assist in the metabolism of our food. Gut health is paramount because the microbiome affects gut-brain communication.

Epigenetics and Alzheimer's Disease and Dementia

Even if you have been dealt a bad hand genetically, you can reshuffle the deck with your epigenetics. That is, by the choices you make regarding diet and lifestyle that ultimately determine the outcome of your health. Both my parents experienced diabetes and had Alzheimer's disease as they progressed in age. These are due primarily, or in part, to plaque accumulation formed by protein deposits in the brain from animal products. The plaque blocks the capillaries, impeding the flow of oxygenated blood to the vital tissues. The animals that we kill are killing us.

Bioaccumulation

Biopsies of fat and muscle tissue of several persons show the same toxins found in the foods they eat are present in their tissues. This is due to the bioaccumulation of toxins. For instance, smaller fish show small percentages of toxins, but larger fish that eat smaller fishes show larger percentages of toxins in their flesh.

Diabetes 2

Working long hours with little or no rest caused me to start gaining weight slowly just before 9/11. When I went to my doctor, I was diagnosed as prediabetic. My naturopathic doctor explained to me that while the high carbs and sweets I was eating contributed to and exacerbated my weight gain, the real cause was something more subtle.

Correlation Is not Always Causation

When I took my parents to their geriatric doctor, he often mentioned to me that they were becoming insulin resistant, and higher doses of insulin would be required to keep their blood sugar in the normal range. Furthermore, I was told that this condition would never be healed or reversed. I asked the doctor why, but never got a satisfactory explanation. The carbs and sugars we consume are supposed to be converted to glucose and absorbed in the liver and muscles. When we are young, this occurs quiet readily since the cell walls are free of years and decades of plaque buildup. This explains why kids who eat as much sugar and candies as adults typically don't develop diabetes 2.

Research found that the walls of the cells can be blocked by accumulation similar to the arterial blockage from proteinaceous deposits that cause heart attacks. It becomes difficult for the glucose to leave the blood and be absorbed in the muscle cells since the cell walls are largely impenetrable to the glucose molecules. This plaque is mainly connected to the animal products we consume. The result is excessive blood sugar. The pancreas is forced to produce more and more insulin in the attempt to decrease the sugar in the blood. This is classic insulin-resistance and results in the pancreas being overworked and exhausted. Eventually, the pancreas is unable to produce insulin efficiently.

But the situation can be changed and diabetes 2 avoided. Once I rested my digestive system by doing intermittent fasting and eating mainly water-based foods, my prediabetic condition went away as the cellular plaque in my muscles and organs broke up and were eliminated.

Leaky Gut

Leaky Gut is a condition in which the lining of the intestinal walls is broken. Whenever this happens, the waste material and bacteria which are the product of digestion leaks through the broken walls and enter the blood stream. This could contaminate the blood stream, causing various kinds of illnesses.

Living microorganisms are found inside the digestive tracks of humans and animals, including insects, called the microbiome. These microorganisms have an important role in physiology. They promote digestion and control immunity. A disruption of this vital microbiome system can result in unrest and imbalance of many body functions. This system needs regular rest, especially if it has been disrupted, to return to normal. Overprocessed food with lots of oil can cause the microbiome to get off balance.

The gut microbiome likes to feed on fiber. In the absence of sufficient fiber, they will start feeding on the gut and break down the walls of the gut. This will cause the gut to leak and allow other particles that should normally be excreted to get into the bloodstream instead.

Fruits have prebiotics the gut microbiome uses to produce probiotics, which are the micronutrients food that your body really needs. Probiotics are essential to maintaining a healthy gut microbiome.

Monthly Menstrual Cramps

I asked one of my clients to do an experiment after she mentioned to me that she suffered from monthly menstrual cramps for several days every month. I asked her to give the digestive system some rest by going on a limited water-based fasting regiment for a month and see if the cramps remain. She would do apple cider vinegar or lemon juice with distilled water and honey for breakfast. For lunch she would have a full garden salad. She would then allow her system to rest for about twenty hours before repeating the process the next day. After the month, the pain was significantly reduced, so she continued with a similar diet of water-based foods with reduced oils. The following months, she experienced no cramps and significantly reduced menstrual flow.

Endocrinologist Dr. Neal Bernard, explained the reason for the cramps. He said the animal-based products typically contain animal hormones, which when added to human hormones, cause excess human female hormones like estrogen to be produced. In turn, this causes an excessive buildup of the uterine walls. While buildup is a normal process that occurs monthly in preparation for fetal development, it gets torn down if pregnancy does not occur. But if this buildup gets excessive, it result in massive a teardown in the form of monthly pain or cramps. A normal amount of buildup causes a normal amount of teardown, which does not result in excessive cramps.

So we see how when the body gets rest from the aggravating products, it will return to homeostasis and proper, painless functioning.

Tips

Control glucose levels at the input (eating) and output (exercise).

Reduce or eliminate animal products from your diet.

Reduce high carbs and sugar.

Exercise a few times per week.

Hydrating the colon through colonics may be helpful, especially if you are constipated.

Fasting will allow the body to break up the plaques in the cell walls.

Sleep for 7 to 9 hours per day. Sleep deprivation can induce a diabetic condition as the muscles become unable to dispose of the excess blood sugar.

Case Study

A woman in New Jersey had diabetes 2 and was fifty pounds overweight. She was on thirteen medications for various conditions and could only walk using a walker. She fasted and ate vegetables only for two weeks, after which her doctor took her off all medications, and she was able to put down her walker. Using these same techniques of fasting and resting the digestive system, I was able to completely reverse and eliminate diabetes 2 and eczema.

1.4 Life in Motion

> Emotion is created by motion. Whatever you're feeling right now is related to how you're using your body.
>
> —Tony Robbins

Motionlessness implies lifelessness. For the body to be properly rested, it must be properly exercised so that the blood can be properly oxygenated and flow through the body. If I exercise when my body is tired or toxic, I would be destroying my muscles instead of building them up. All muscles and joints need to be stretched and flexed or twisted on a regular basis to function properly. If you do not use it, you will lose it.

The lymphatic system is a system of tube-like vessels which provides a way for the body to drain itself of cellular and metabolic toxic debris. Unlike the cardiovascular system, the lymphatic system does not have a pump. Lymphatic fluid is only moved by exercise. Exercise also releases endorphins that improve one's mood as well as cardiovascular health. Stretching of the muscles promotes joint health for balance and mobility. Strong muscles support joints by keeping off some of the load on them.

Movement provides about 90 percent of the stimulation that the brain needs. The spine has several hundred muscles over two to three layers whose movements provide indirect stimulation of the brain. Exercise is one of the best ways to stimulate the brain, and the body in general. Even though exercise stresses the body in some ways, it makes the body more adaptable to the stress. Whenever we exercise, we are putting a kind of stress on the body. The body senses this stress and processes it the same way it would if this were an attack. The survival instincts kick in and the body builds up resistance to make it stronger.

Posture

Physical movements and motions determine one's feelings or emotions. Research found that whenever we stand erect or take on the superhero posture, our immune systems are boosted, and stress hormones, such as cortisol, levels decrease.

We should also try to maintain proper posture because it helps keep the skeletal system properly aligned for weight distribution on various joints. The center of gravity of the body is in the lower back, and as millions of people worldwide suffer from backache, we need to exercise the muscles and joints that keep this region properly functioning.

Exercise improves many of the same biomarkers that fasting improves. For example, if you keep one of your arms in a sling for two months, without any motion in its joints, do you think that arm will function normally after you release the sling? Of course not. The muscles will fossilize and seize. We need to keep all our joints and muscles moving to keep them working optimally.

You may think that you need expensive gym memberships and advanced equipment to exercise effectively. But just doing simple movements on a regular basis can be very beneficial to the body. Exercises like squats, jumping jacks, walking or jogging in place or in a park, boxing in the air, push-ups on an incline or on the floor, Pilates, and yoga are among the ways to keep the body in optimal condition with as little as a few minutes per day.

Eye Exercise

This exercise provides much-need exercise to the badly underexercised eyes, helping to improve circulation and remove mucus and cellular deposit buildups.

There are three parts to this exercise: rolling the eyes, tapping around the eyes, and massaging the eyes. This entire exercise can be repeated several times throughout the day until you see changes in your ability to see smaller things more clearly. It is a great idea to lightly rinse the face with pure water before and after you finish all these eye exercises.

Rolling the Eyes

This involves keeping the head steady and rolling both eyes to the extreme left and then holding it for several seconds. Then do the same for extreme right. Next, look down as far as possible, and hold the gaze for a few seconds. Then look all the way up, and hold for a few seconds. Finally, attempt to look at the nose with both eyes. and hold for a few seconds before releasing.

Tapping the Eyes

Use a fingers to lightly tap around the eyes and then on the top, sides, and just below the eyes. Use the left hand to tap the left eye and the right hand to tap the right eye.

Massaging the Eyes

With both eyes are closed, use the index and middle fingers to gently wipe the top of each eyelid from the side closest to the nose to the side farthest from the nose. Do the same for below the eyes. Then wipe down the sides from top to bottom.

Marathon

As I began to heal from the trauma of 9/11, I gave up certain devitalizing food and my toxic lifestyle. I started to run and exercise more, which in turn gave me more energy. I finally decided that I wanted to run in the NYC marathon, so I started to train for it.

The word "marathon" is derived from the name of a Greek city, Marathon. Legend has it that a young man ran from Marathon to Athens to announce the victory of the battle at Marathon.

Exercise not only build our physical muscles, it also builds our mental muscles. Yes, it allows us to be live longer. Even though I am super-interested in longevity, I don't know the exact length of our lives on earth. When we set a goal to exercise, we are saying to ourselves that we can set goals and achieve them. We are saying that we are in control of our lives. And it allows us to set and achieve other goals, like spiritual and financial goals. The results that we experience from exercise, such as doing more reps or lifting heavier weights, give us confidence that we can expand our lives in other areas. It incentivizes us to transform other areas of our lives and lets us know that we can change any areas of our lives. We discover that we are not at the mercy of our environments, which have limited control over our lives. We are the masters of our destinies. Working on our bodies is the beginning of working on our mental proactive muscles.

One other good thing about exercise in general, and running in particular, is that it pushes blood to the brain to keep us healthy. What's the mechanism behind this? When we run, our feet pound whatever surface we're running on. Typically, when an object that contains particles, like a jar of sand and water, is pounded on a hard surface, the expectation is that gravity and momentum will cause the particles or fluid to settle in the lower parts of the object. Likewise, the expectation is that the blood in the body will move from the top of the head to settle in the lower extremities when one's feet pound the pavement. This does, in fact, happen; the blood does move from our heads to our lower extremities.

However, by natural adaptation, there is a valve in the upper part of the body that pushes blood to our brains whenever our feet pound the pavement. For example, in the case where we are running from a predator, the brain never runs out of blood when we need it most to think and escape as blood is settled to the lower extremities. Otherwise, the brain would run out of blood, and one would faint and be overtaken by a predator. So running, having our feet pound the pavement, makes our brains work better. However, this exercise must be balanced with the condition of our feet, leg joints, and muscles.

Running requires proper gear. Shoes must have adequate cushioning and padding and be designed for surfaces like grass that are not too hard so that it will not damage the ankle, knee, hip, or back joints. I found a trampoline to be very useful and easier on the body while achieving similar results. Lying on your back while doing certain exercises is also helpful. Please consult your doctor for specific exercise regimens. And start off gradually and slowly as you build up to regular pace.

Daily Core Exercises

Here is an illustration of various targeted exercises that will allow you to stay in homeostasis and enjoy better rest. These exercises are mainly for the back and abdominals, which involve twisting left and right; bending forward, backward, and sideways; lateral stretching, which can be done with the head up, hanging from a bar, with the head down, or hanging at an angle using specialized equipment—if approved by your doctor. Rest must be earned through exercise like these and more.

Daily Stretching & Exercising Routine

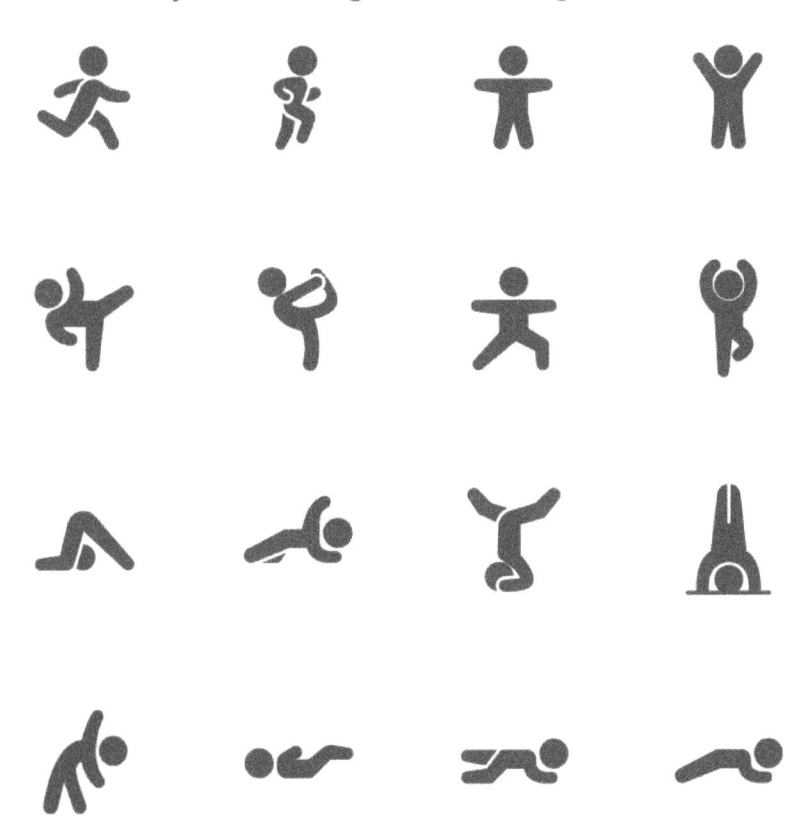

1.5 Water-Based Feasting

> The best of all medicines is resting and fasting.
>
> —Benjamin Franklin.

Fasting is resting the entire digestive system for a period when they can be revitalized. It is not starving. When we put away food and do not eat for a time, the body uses up the stored nutrients in the liver and burns excess fat, lowering bad cholesterol and reducing excessive weight. Ketosis occurs after twenty-four hours of fasting, when the body only burns fat for energy. This is a cleaner and more efficient form of energy. When this happens, you feel better, and you get more mental clarity. Human growth hormone (HGH), which is used to repair the cell instead of dividing it, increases significantly when food is absent. Autophagy occurs during fasting, when the body uses energy that is normally used for digestion to recycle old and broken cell components and to replace malformed and cancerous cells. This process removes the chemicals and pesticides that get lodged in the cells from garden vegetables. Stem cell production occurs in the bone marrow and can be used to completely make new organs.

The body consists of mostly water. The brain, heart, lungs, skin, muscles, and kidneys consist of a high percentage of water. Even the bones have a substantial percentage of water.

According to US Geological Survey, water serves a number of essential functions to keep us all going:

- A vital nutrient to the life of every cell, it acts first as a building material.
- It regulates our internal body temperature by sweating and respiration.
- The carbohydrates and proteins that our bodies use as food are metabolized and transported by water in the bloodstream.
- It assists in flushing waste mainly through urination.
- It acts as a shock absorber for brain, spinal cord, and fetus.
- It forms saliva.
- It lubricates joints.

Different foods consist of different amounts of water. Since the food we eat will ultimately be assimilated in our bodies, the higher the water content of the food, the less stress these foods put on the body for digestion, and the more the body stays in a state of homeostasis. Foods that are produced by Mother Nature have a higher water content than commercially produced foods. Additionally, foods produced by Mother Nature are less likely to have preservatives that negatively affect our biological systems, especially when organically grown. Plant-based foods are also a primary source of nutrients. Animal-based foods, however, are secondary sources of nutrients in the sense that the animals consume the plant nutrients and store it in their bodies, and then humans eat the animal product. One can easily see that the loss of nutrients and toxic accumulation are more likely with secondary, animal-based products. What I am saying is that animal products have a higher probability of containing environmental toxins compared to plant-based foods. I am not necessarily saying it is altogether bad for us or that we should not eat animal products.

Foods that are highly processed typically have a low water content and low fiber. Most also are high in salt, sugar, and saturated oils.

Since the body is made up of more than 80 percent water, the quality of water we drink is essential. After all, it will ultimately become the building blocks of our bodies.

Here are some foods high in water content:

- Watermelon
- Apples
- Pears
- Peaches
- Cucumbers
- Tomatoes
- Celery
- Lettuce
- Oranges

Foods that are water-based put less stress on the digestive system. And the less stress placed on the digestive system by the foods we consume, the more efficient these foods will be in healing the body, and the less effort the body will have to exert to eliminate toxins and repair the body.

Are the foods that appeal to you water-based and go with your body, thereby naturally supporting it? Or are they so different from your body that your body will spend a lot of resources to eliminate them?

Distilled Water

Pure distilled water puts the least amount of stress on the body. It also has the added benefit of removing toxins from the organs through the process of osmosis. Through osmatic pressure created by pure water, toxins diffuse into the water and are eliminated through channels like the kidney and skin. Conversely, toxin from foods can be defused into the cells.

There are many levels of water purity based on the filtration system used. Some filtration systems allow some substances to escape. Distilled water is the purest. The distillation process involves evaporating water, leaving all impurities behind. Water is the only substance to evaporate at 100 degrees; other substances, like alcohols, will evaporate before the water reaches that temperature and escape into the atmosphere. For commercial or residential distillation purposes, the now-distilled water can be passed through a carbon filter so dissolved gasses can be removed. The distillation process is created by nature and has been used the world over for centuries before industrialization and the development of complex filtration plants. This is the same process by which rainwater is used for domestic purposes all over the world. The sun evaporates the streams, the vapor condenses as clouds, and then the clouds precipitate and fall back to earth as rain.

Water generally symbolizes cleansing; it has a frequency. Water responds to thoughts and words. The water in our bodies can respond to gratitude and kindness to create healing.

Vital Life-Giving Force

The body is largely self-healing. That is, given the right conditions and resources, it will heal itself if it is not obstructed. This healing mechanism is the result of the natural life-giving force that will always attempt to self-correct any damage as best as it can. For example, if you cut your finger, you do not need to tell the body to do anything. It will automatically start to send repair material and other elements to the finger to keep away any other organisms that may try to enter the body through that area. Healing has less to do with something in a bottle and more to do with the innate life force. The medicine can, however, assist in reducing bacterial or toxins so the immune system can do its job better.

This innate life force is at work in our subconscious minds even when we are asleep. It is responsible for all body functions, including digestion, assimilation, respiration, repair, and blood sugar level even when we are asleep. We could never consciously calculate the increased amount of sugar needed to be released in the blood to maintain the body temperature, for example.

Whenever there is toxic overload, life-giving forces that normally repair the body are first diverted to remove toxins. This is like a situation where we want to bring new groceries into our home, but if a kitchen is filled with garbage or debris from yesterday, no more new and good stuff can be brought in until we clear out the old stuff and make room for the new. Notice how just after a meal we feel drowsy? This is because vital forces in the form of blood are diverted from the brain and limbs to the digestive organs to break down the food. Therefore, less energy is left over for activities.

After 9/11, I experienced how this life force cleared my eyes, brain fog, and skin condition; cleansed the liver; and restored digestive juices to reduce blood sugar, but only after I was able to go into a deep rest using meditation, fasting, and other techniques.

Breakfast: The Fast That Gets Broken

Everyone fasts. A limited version of resting the digestive system—aka fasting—occurs daily when we go to bed at night, not eating anything during our sleep. Obviously, we cannot eat and sleep at the same time, unless we are sleep walking and sleep-eating. (Yes, there is such a thing.) We then wake up and eat our first meal in the morning to break the fast, hence the term "breakfast."

Resting the entire digestive system for a period in order to be revitalized is not starving. Any method of reducing food intake—like intermittent fasting, keto diet, mindful eating, low-carb, and so on—that results in resting the digestive system provides some benefits. The longer the resting period, the better and more beneficial, generally speaking, but it should be done within limits. If I am in a state of great health, then a regular daily fasting of about sixteen to twenty hours can maintain my body in optimal condition. According to Dr. Jason Fung, one of the leading experts in fasting, this can be achieved by skipping the morning routine, since when we just wake up, we are still energized. Then, have a full-course meal sometime between 11 a.m. and 3 p.m., so we are still not hungry by the time we go to bed.

The study "Effects of Intermittent Fasting on Health, Aging and Disease," by Rafael de Cabo, PhD and Mark P. Mattson, PhD, was published on March 5, 2020, in the *New England Journal of Medicine* (*NEJM*). The *NEJM* is one of the most prestigious scholarly journals in the world. Articles must be thoroughly validated before they are published. The authors were very thorough and articulate. They studied animals before it was validated in humans. Two groups were used in the study. The first group ate all their meals once or twice per day. The second group had the same amount of food, but it was spread throughout the day. Those in the first group showed better health indicators at the end, showing that when you eat is as important as what you eat.

In another study, women who reduced their calories while eating throughout the day did not do as well as those who had the same calorie reduction but limited their eating to once or twice a day. While both groups experienced weight loss, the last group had reduced waist size and better insulin response, and so on.

There were metabolic switches when the body was rested, which causes the unclogging of the body. The results included weight loss and reductions in cancer, asthma, breathing problems, arthritis, joint inflammation, and heart and memory problems.

Benefits of Fasting

Whenever we reduce food intake for any period, several phenomenal beneficial processes take place. Nature is simple yet supple.

> *Lowering of bad cholesterol:* Our bodies use up stored nutrients in the liver and burn up excess fat to lower bad cholesterol and reduce excessive weight.
>
> *Lowering of blood sugar:* The blood sugar is used for energy. This allows the body to have a better insulin response. Metabolic flexibility occurs when one form of energy is low, and the body seemlessly turns to another source of energy.
>
> *Ketosis:* This typically occurs if the resting of the digestive system is extended to twenty hours and beyond for days. When insulin output for food is minimal, the body burns only fat for energy. When sugar is low, the body turns to fat-burning and produces ketones. This is a cleaner and more efficient form of energy. It makes you feel better and gives you a sharper mind.
>
> All foods—including sugars, fats, carbohydrates, and proteins—are converted into a common substance called adenosine triphosphate (ATP) that the body can use for energy. This is the only form of energy the body can use.

After eighteen to twenty-four hours of fasting, drinking water only, the glucose level goes down and the ketones, HGH, and insulin levels begin to go up, which causes the amount of autophagy to increase as well. As the fast is continued for another two to six days or more, these factors continue to increase.

Supply and Demand Diagram: Ketones vs. Sugar over 120 Hours of Fasting

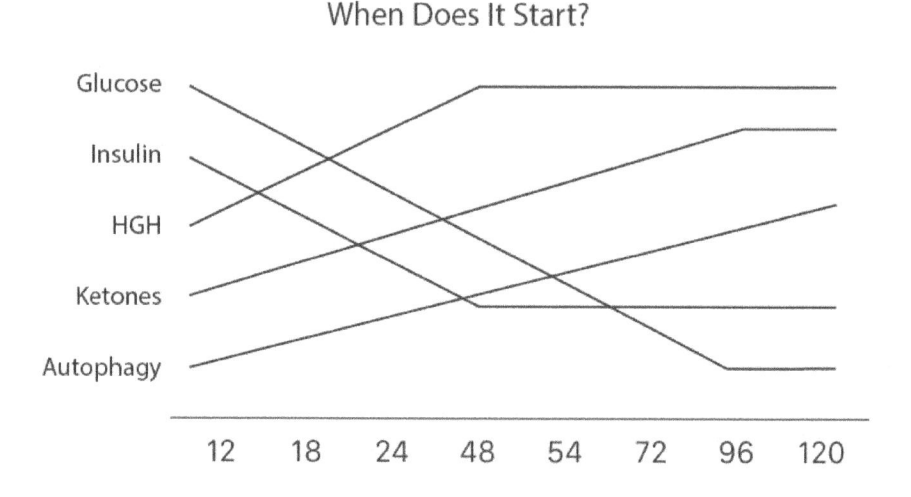

When Does It Start?

Mental Clarity: Existentially, whenever an animal lacks food, it does not die instantly but starts to hunt for food, so the mind needs to be sharper and to work more efficiently in order to find food very fast in order to survive.

HGH: Human growth hormone, which is used to repair cells instead of dividing them, increases significantly when food is absent.

Autophagy: During prolonged digestive rest, the body uses energy that is normally used for digestion to recycle old and broken cell components and replace malformed cells. These processes are possible only because the resources of the body that are normally used for regular digestion are redirected to executing recycling.

Weight Loss: As the body uses up the stored sugar, it begins to metabolize the excess fat for energy. Biopsies of human fat cells show that they are prime storage sites for salts, oils, and other toxins digested and absorbed through the skin. These toxins are then removed via the excretory channels.

Stem Cell: These are the originator cells, baby cells that go to create other organs. The body's ability to maintain its function is directly related to the number of stem cells in the bloodstream to perform natural cell repair and renewal. Stem cells are naturally generated in increasingly significant levels after days of fasting. Stem cells are very costly to be administered artificially, and it is less than 1 percent effective when administered exogenously. However, when the body produces them endogenously, the stem cells go to the right areas in the right amounts, naturally repairing damaged cells as they blend in with the biochemistry of the cell.

Babies produce stem cells that are circulated in the mothers' bloodstream via the umbilical cord. These stem cells help to heal and repair the mother's organs. This is done so the baby can have the fittest, healthiest environment to grow in. The baby is taking care of what will take care of it for decades to come.

Circadian-Based Fasting: Stay Hungry

Alan Goldhamer and Jennifer Marano are the founders of TrueNorth Health Center—www.healthpromoting.com—one of the first and largest facilities in the world that specialize in medically supervised water-based fasting. They have overseen thousands of water-based fasts and helped patients radically transform their lives, from ditching medication to overcoming a litany of common but chronic lifestyle diseases.

Objection to any kind of fasting may occur because it may be viewed from a limiting perspective as starvation or cause of hunger headaches. First, fasting, whether overnight or for several weeks, is not starvation. The ingenuity of the body is its ability to store enough food, so we can go for weeks without eating. There is a recorded instance where a person was lost in the woods for many days. When he was discovered and brought to the hospital, it was found that his vital organs—like his heart, brain, gonads, and nervous system—were intact, and the excess fat and waste materials were spent up by the body. Several experiments have been documented in the *NEJM* showing that in fasts lasting several days and even weeks under a medical doctor's supervision, subjects showed very little or no loss of vital organ function. The body is smart and will not destroy vital organs at the first instance of hunger. This is similar to a situation where, if you are cold in your home and are unable to go out and get wood, and you have old, unused furniture in your home, you will burn up the old stuff before you burn the new, expensive furniture.

Second, the so-called hunger pain is due to habit hunger and emotional eating, which are automatic processes based on practice. Habitual eating cycles and the release of toxins are the root cause of hunger pain and urges. Because the body is used to eating at certain times, the body's digestive juices are secreted, hence we get the urge to eat and the feelings of hunger, even though the body could go longer without starving. If we don't eat at that time, the body's energies will go into removing stored toxins from the cells. When these toxins are released in the bloodstream, they cause the headaches. At this point, before the headache gets too severe, some natural fruit juice or organic tea with lemon and honey can be used to dissolve these toxins. They can then be passed through the eliminating channels, and the headache will go away, so you can continue to fast.

I recommend gradually introducing more foods with a higher water content in the routine diet over several days and weeks, and gradually eliminate the foods that have low water content, that is, toxic foods. This will allow the slow release of toxins without the excessive headaches. I will concede that if someone who has never fasted should suddenly go on a fast for several days without the proper guidance, he or she will be challenged. I would not advise undertaking a fast for several days without medical supervision and guidance.

Practical Steps

Here are some practical guidelines to begin fasting for an extended period. Let us say you normally do two or three meals per day. Some people even eat six meals per day—morning, afternoon, and evening snacks—that can overdrive the digestive channels and exhaust the vital life force. A good place to start is to substitute one heavy meal for a lighter one, like a salad, smoothie, or just juice. Then after a week, one meal can be eliminated or substituted for water, so you are down to two meals per day, so your body gets acclimated to the new routine without any withdrawal symptoms. If hunger feelings arise during this time, a glass of water will flush out the toxins and remove any feelings of hunger until the next meal.

The next few weeks, you can do the same for the second meal. By gradual substitution and elimination over several weeks, you can go for days on just water without feeling withdrawal symptoms or pain. The result is that the latent toxins within the cells will be eliminated gradually, and with new habits, we may be able to eat once per day or every other day. You may eventually be able to go several days or weeks without food on just the vital stored energy of the body without feeling hungry or entering starvation. However, any amount of time that you are able to rest the digestive system will benefit the body in some way as vital energy is diverted toward repair rather than digestion. Even resting the digestive system for more than eight hours, say twelve or sixteen or twenty hours per day, on a regular basis can be beneficial.

It is recommended to continue to take vitamins supplements and medications. Children, pregnant or nursing mothers, and people with certain medical conditions should not go for prolonged periods without food. If you have any of the degenerative illnesses, a longer fast may prove more beneficial. In every case, we must consult a medical doctor before making any changes to our diets.

During this time of not eating, it is recommended to engage in some other important activities or hobbies, like painting, writing, volunteering, and meditation – based on your level of health.

A Testimony on Weight Loss and Respiratory Restoration

A seventy-two-year-old friend mentioned he was having some vision issues; there were some dark spots in his field of vision. He also had diabetes 2 and arthritis. His doctor had him on several medications. I gave him some guidance on how he could rest his digestive system by changing his intake to mainly water-based foods initially, and then periodically on water so the vital healing energy of his body could get to work. After a few weeks, he came back to me and said that his doctor took him off all his medications! His blood sugar was normal, the back pain left, and his vision had cleared. The vital life force had removed and flushed out the excessive dead cells from his blood and joints, and it restored the fluids in his eyes. By resting the pancreas, it started to produce the normal amount of insulin. Additionally, he lost the excess weight, his skin was more radiant, and he was able to breathe better when he walked in the park.

Spiritual Cleansing

Sages over the ages have fasted for spiritual and physical benefits. They include leaders from every religious background, such as Moses, Jesus, Socrates, Gandhi, Buddha, and Mohammed. It was seen as a cleansing. We need to be careful about what we eat, but equally important are how and when we eat for it was eating the forbidden fruit that caused our foreparents to lose their standing and driven from the garden of paradise. Also, over the past centuries, various civilizations were forced to fast due to various changes in seasons, war, and so on.

Emotional Eating

It's not what you eat, it is what's eating you. What's eating you? Do we eat to satisfy some emotional craving? Or do we eat to satisfy real physical hunger? If we have real emotional needs that are not met, then we will tend to binge on junk foods that adversely affect our health. We will then pass on these and other habits on to our kids. By extension also, if our kids are fed the same mindset of poverty and lack, they grow up and have lives that are limiting. So that is why we see that poverty and wealth are generational.

Tips for Proper Eating

- First thing in the morning, squeeze a lemon in a glass of warm water or apple cider vinegar and drink it.
- For breakfast, I typically have fruit or vegetable juices, or raw fruits based on the season.
- The heaviest meal is when the sun is highest in the sky. This is when the digestive juices are at their maximum. This meal is largely water-based food from natural plants, which can provide a balance of protein, carbohydrates, and fiber.
- Try to reduce animal-based food or overprocessed refined flour, sugar, rice, and milk.

Natural Foods That Detoxify

Garlic
Aloe vera
Ginger
Lemon
Turmeric
Dandelion
Beet
Milk thistle
Artichoke extract
L-cysteine
Alfalfa
Seaweed extract
Macca

1.6 Breathing in the Life Force

> Life isn't about how many breaths you take, but it's about those moments that take your breath away.
>
> —Will Smith

Pollutants from the WTC severely affected the breathing of thousands of people in the days and months after the attack. Breathing-related illnesses like asthma, sleep apnea, pneumonia, and now COVID-19 are spiraling out of control. Breathing properly can increase our lungs' capacities and efficiency.

The word "breath" is derived from "pneuma," which is connected to air. When we stop breathing, we are dead. The expression, "Catch my breath," or, "Take a breather," means to rest. For a healthy life, we should be breathing at about twelve breaths per minute. However, the average American breathes about eighteen times per minute.

We need to do nasal rather than mouth breathing with a complete exhalation to expel all the CO_2 before we take in a full breath of oxygen. The nasal passage has filters and membranes to moisten and enhance the quality of the air that reaches the lungs. Overbreathing can be caused by several things, including breathing disorders or panic attacks. Proper breathing lowers heart rate and blood pressure.

The diaphragm is a biomechanical pump that creates movements for the lungs and, in turn, air flow. Additionally, it provides movement of lymph fluid and sends signals to the brain. When we perceive that we are under attack, our breathing temporarily becomes fast and shallow. This takes oxygen away from our vital organs and puts it in the musculoskeletal system for flight or fight.

We heal when we slow down the mind and body when we meditate. Whenever we take our focus off the externals, such as social media, and focus on the breath going through our beings, we are refreshed and enlivened. When we take our minds off past problems or future dreams and direct our energies internally, we are revitalized.

The word "hallelujah" is the same in all languages. It represents the breath of the super-consciousness in all humans. Whenever we stop breathing our bodies will expire as the animating force departs.

Breath helps to pull the energies of the body from the belly, or the lower centers of the body, to the heart and brain. When we are scared, our breaths become irregular and imbalanced. Fear and anxiety overwhelm and tighten our breathing, weakening our immune system. Notice how our breathing changes by becoming freer after we experience something pleasurable.

If we find two animals in the wild, and one is breathing heavily, and the other is breathing slowly and deeply, which one would you conclude is at rest? Which one would you think is in danger and being hunted?

The perception of danger sends signals along the vagus nerves that activate the sympathetic system which prepares the body for flight or fight. While the parasympathetic system moves the body out of stress and back to calmness. Men and women in the military are trained to take deep breaths, to activate the parasympathetic system, especially during a crisis, such as when bombs are going off and shots are being fired, so that they can pull the blood back to the frontal cortex for better focus and decision-making and not panic. As we slow our breathing, it reduces panic and anxiety attacks. Navy Seal breathe rhythmically before a mission to activate the parasympathetic system.

Aromatherapy

When we are anxious, the part of the brain that is active is connected to smell. So aromatherapy can be helpful. Aromatherapy uses natural oils and plant extracts mixed with water. When this mixture is heated, the scent of it can be very calming as it spreads in a room. Certain scents, like jasmine and lavender, can be especially helpful to breath in.

Air Pollution

Many cities of our nation and around the world are affected by toxic air pollution from chemicals used in or produced by manufacturing plants and transportation. Occasionally, these factories and refineries have accidents and fires that result in massive amounts of toxic smoke being blown in the air close to residences. This air is inhaled by residences, and they develop chronic illnesses, sometimes years later. These chemicals include organic and sulfur derivatives. Recent US administrations have rolled back the protection provided by the Environmental Protection Agency (EPA). And the country withdrew from the global G7 alliance, the top seven countries that govern regulations regarding air and environmental conditions.

Air purifiers with carbon filters or water-based filtration systems may be of some value to clear some of these pollutants from the air.

Breathing Exercises

One of the quickest ways to refresh and slow our breathing is to take three deep breaths with six seconds in and six seconds out. This exercise can be repeated as amny times as needed throughout the day, especially when you feel anxious or stressed.

2

MIND

We essentially live in an environment created by our thoughts. Despite what is going on around us, we need to envision a future based on our true passions and feel the emotions of having and living those passions. We do not need to wait for our gifts to feel good. If we stop worrying about past setbacks and start to feel the love, our bodies and minds will move from a place of disease to one of rest and healing. Worrying is looking back at the past and replaying or reliving the negative experiences and imagining the worst-case scenarios. On the other hand, vision looks forward at the infinite possibility of good things that can happen. We should seek to pre-play the positive instead of replaying the negative. There was a successful football team that, at the beginning of each season, made the entire team, including the rookies, watch videos of past victories and feel the excitement. This played an important role in the victories they achieved regularly.

2.1 Emotionally Balanced

> Strong emotions such as passion and bliss are indications that you're connected to Spirit, or "inspired," if you will. When you're inspired, you activate dormant forces, and the abundance you seek in any form comes streaming into your life.
>
> —Wayne Dyer

Flight or Fight

Whenever any living organism is under attack, it goes into a state of fight or flight. This engages the sympathetic nervous system that throws the body out of homeostasis, relaxation, and ease. For instance, if you are being chased by a saber-toothed tiger, you will need all your energy to escape and survive. In survival mode, the body sends most of the blood away from the internal organs to the external limbs and systems for optimal fight or flight. During this time, some of the organs affected are the eyes, which will dilate for optimal vision and focus; the heart rate will increase as it sends extra oxygenated blood to the limbs; and the stress hormones, like cortisol, and breathing increase significantly. This is a most stressful time for the body because resources normally meant to nourish and maintain the body are redirected for escape.

Emotional Turmoil

The body does not distinguish between an external stressor, such as a tiger, and an internal one coming from the mind. Just like being in a state of physical distress, when we are in a state of emotional distress, the mind similarly activates the brain to send signals to the various body systems. For instance, in our day-to-day activities, if we perceive any kind of threat in our environment, the mind can trigger the body to go into that state. If we have a conflict or argument with a family member or coworker, if we hit traffic on our way to work or school, this state can be triggered. The body does not know the difference between a real and an imagined predator; it experiences the same primal response to an attack. Living in this state for a short time is sometimes necessary, but to live in this survival state constantly is extremely destructive.

Expanded Focus

Whenever we find ourselves in the survival state, we can get back to the steady, restful state of equilibrium by shifting our consciousnesses. For example, this can be done by slowly inhaling and then slowly exhaling. Most important, we need to take time every morning, before we get out of bed and out and about, to meditate and enter a place of gratitude so that we can get ready for the day. This time should be before we pick up our cell phones or devices and start checking our emails, text messages, or social media. We should always seek to be in a place of homeostasis and not dependent on the external events to control our internal moods and emotions. When we pick up our cell phones first thing in the morning, we are training our proactive minds to be weaker and to follow other people's agendas instead of setting out on our own agendas. Social media can be addictive because it lights up the dopamine or reward centers, causing us to want more. Extreme addictions can lead to depressions and a downward spiral of life.

As we meditate, we train the mind to move from a narrow focus to a broader one. This can help the body to enter a state of relaxation. When we are attacked by a tiger, for instance, our focus becomes acute as we seek to identify the exact location and speed of the predator, and more so as we look for a clear path to escape. During this time, we would not care much about how beautiful the meadow is or how blue the sky is.

In the stressful state, we focus on the negatives because we need to remember details about the attack so that if the predator should show up again, we can recognize and avoid that negative situation to survive. This is a natural existential reaction.

Paranoia and PTSD

Like many others, I experienced PTSD after the attacks on the WTC. Whenever I entered the city and saw a plane when I looked up—even if it is far away—I would get that tight feeling in my stomach. Before 9/11, when we came out of the subway, we would look up to see the WTC towers and get our bearings. But after the towers fell, we were kind of lost for a while, until we found another reference point on which we could catch our bearings. This is symbolic to what the country was going through in the moments and days and weeks after the attack.

Post-traumatic stress disorder—PTSD—occurs when someone experiences something that is emotionally impacting. The mind takes a snapshot of it and stores it as memory. This event causes the body to go through a rush of hormones that prepares it for fight or flight. If in the future that person experiences anything similar or related to the original event, the mind will go back to experiencing the event all over again. The body will go through that same emotional response. Even though the actual event is past and gone, the body will relive that event. This is important because the organism needs to remember the bad stuff that threatened its survival in the past and be ready to defend itself against it or something similar in the future. Therefore, anything that even remotely reminds the organism of the past trauma could trigger that response. We should not let the external circumstances determine our internal states.

When a person experiences unrest for a prolonged period, for example if he or she has been in a war zone and experienced trauma—such as bombings, land mines, and shootings—the person with PTSD may expect to be attacked or blown up with every step taken. This puts the mind in a state of permanent hyperalertness and unrest. In this state of paranoia, anything that closely resembles the original condition can trigger that response. Loud noises or the appearance of any sharp edges, for example, can remind the person of the original incident. One of the best ways to break the habit of paranoia is the daily practice of visualization and meditation combined with gratitude for the future success.

Notice that the rehearsal of the event puts the body in that same emotional and chemical state. However, that emotional association to the traumatic event can be broken by creating a different set of associations over time through some very specific meditations.

Studies show that neural pathways within the body that gets built through constant repetition will readily allow certain thoughts, feelings, and abilities to exist and flow through it, like a river that consistently runs down a certain path. This is what is incorrectly labelled as "muscle memory," when in fact it should be called "neuron memory."

The way to prevent these negative thoughts and feelings from overcoming the individual is to divert energy and thinking into new neural pathways, allowing new routes to be built that readily allow the flow of neurons that, in turn, create new thoughts and feelings. The more a person thinks back on past traumas, the deeper the PTSD is entrenched.

Resting and Restoring the Mind through Visualization

During my illness, I spent many days visualizing different parts of my body being healed. I would lie quietly on my back for half an hour each morning, before I got up to do anything, and imagine my sinuses being cleared through each breath that I took. I imagined my breath flowing from my feet into my stomach, up into my heart, and up to my head, clearing and removing toxins from my skin, eyes, and other organs as it went.

Visualization is a very powerful technique that has been used by many professionals and even athletes and movie stars. One Olympic gold medalist said that the key to her winning was visualization because it instilled the neurological and physiological conditions necessary to accomplish the tasks. The more detailed we can visualize, the better will be our results.

The practice of visualization and meditation will start to break down old nerve connections and make new nerve connections in the brain. With these new connections, we can experience new emotions that cause the breaking of old habits.

A study was done on a group of students who were learning to play the guitar by practicing scales for about thirty minutes every day. The students were divided into two groups: those who physically played with their fingers and those who only rehearsed the scales in their minds. All the students had brain scans at the beginning and at the end of the study. It was found that both groups of students grew new brain neurons in response to the practice. One could not distinguish between either group of students based on the brain scans.

Vibrational States of the Mind and Programming

You don't have to be a neurosurgeon to understand the brain. There is so much to learn about the brain to use it to its full potential. The brain has nerve cells that produce electrical signals with distinctive patterns called brain wave patterns. These waves have very distinct vibrational frequencies based on our emotional states, moods, thoughts, activities, consciousnesses, and biochemistries. They can be measured by external instruments. There are basically four states of the consciousness based on the vibrational frequency, ranging from high frequency to low: beta, alpha, theta, and delta.

State	Frequency (in Hz)	Consciousness	Alertness
Beta	13–40	Fully Conscious	Fully Alert
Alpha	7–13	Subconscious	Relaxed
Theta	4–7	Unconscious	Trancelike
Delta	0–4	Superconscious	Deep Sleep

In beta, the mind is busy with day-to-day activities as you are conscious. In high beta, the mind is extremely alert; for example, if you are hunted by a predator or have a major academic test.

In alpha, you go into a deeper state of relaxation, and brain wave frequency is lowered.

In theta, you are in a trancelike state that produces dreams, intuition, and creativity.

And in delta, you are just waking from sleep or just falling off to sleep. In this state, the mind is very receptive to new information.

Heal from Your Scars and not Your Wounds

A few weeks before I was terminated from my job in the WTC, I had a major emotional breakdown as my relationship with my life partner became upended. This was due at least in part to my physical health, and in turn, it affected my psychological and emotional health. I was working long hours and not getting enough restful sleep, and that caused me to be edgy. There were constant arguments and flare-ups between us, so I contemplated moving on or moving away to avoid conflicts and confrontations. Even when my wife and I spoke over the phone regarding the kids, it was so tense. I discovered firsthand that emotional instability affects my health because it drives up my blood pressure and causes anxiety.

Also, my emotional instability was affecting my relationship with the people who did not hurt me. If we don't heal when we are hurt, we will bleed on people who did not hurt us. Many months after I had rested and relaxed my mind, body, and spirit, I experienced tranquility and restorative healing, so I was reconciled to my family. I was only able to heal my family after my emotional wounds were healed and had become scars. My scars are now a badge of honor of what I have been through and therefore, my ability to help others to heal.

What makes you happy? What do you do for fun? What makes you want to take on the world. Emotional health is a major contributor to overall well-being even if you eat right. You must move away from the sympathetic states (flight or flight), which are created by anger, hurt, and disillusionment. Strong emotions cause the activation of certain physiological processes, just like deep happiness can trigger laughter, and extreme sadness can trigger tears. Our levels of excitement about our healings can significantly influence our recoveries.

What hinders the ability to come into abundance of health and peace? Are you properly equipped to provide the quality service that will allow you to come into your purpose? Fear, guilt, criticism, and anger must be properly dealt with for us to step into purpose. Fear makes us petrified or frozen, and impedes our movements, which are manifested in our joints. Guilt tells us, "Hit me over my head. If you don't hit me, I will hit myself," and anger says, "You hurt me," and it is seen in our breathing. Criticism affects the flexibility of our joints. Like Tarzan, you cannot grab the next branch until you let go of the last one. The thing that saves you can hurt you if you hold on to it for too long. Catch the next wave because the current one is going to die.

Here are five steps to healing an emotion once you have identified it in your being:

>Step 1: Take responsibility for your emotion.
>Step 2: Express the emotion through journaling.
>Step 3: Release the emotion through exercise, movements, or music.
>Step 4: Talk to an emphatic listener.
>Step 5: Treat yourself to something you love—massage, gift, snack.

2.2 Musication: Music as Medicine

> Music is the soundtrack of our life.
>
> —Dr. Joe Despanza

The word "musication" is a cross between music and medication. It is believed that music is a form of medication. It has helped to heal stroke patients and calm the mind. Research shows that music produces opioids in the brain that help to calm the body. For centuries, music has been used to heal princes and paupers alike. Music is the wind beneath our wings on which the soul takes flight into bliss and joy, transporting us on its wings back to past experiences of happy or sad memories.

Do you know the feeling you get when you hear certain music that you cannot resist dancing or moving to? My first exposure to music and singing was in church. We had some long services in Jamaica in those days. My parents were in the church and mandated us to go to church for Sunday school at 9 a.m. for an hour. After that, we would attend regular church service for three to four hours. Then we would go back for evangelistic service at 7 p.m. for another three or four hours. Then we would be back for youth service on Monday nights, missionary service on Wednesday nights, and choir practice Friday nights. As a kid, I always wondered why church services were so long, but I guess it filled the time and kept us out of trouble since TV and the internet was not what it is today.

In most of our services, we sang, and there was a band consisting of a guitar, a drum set, tambourines, and cymbals. When the music started, the pastor or deacons would start clapping vigorously to the song, and many of the people from the church would start dancing and skipping in the spirit, often knocking over chairs and benches.

Outside of church, we were able to hear music on the radio from the one or two stations we could pick up. We had a grainy, black-and-white TV, and music videos were broadcast at certain times, especially in the summer. Our parents did not want us to listen to secular music because it would be a bad influene. However, when my parents were away at work or gone to the store, my bigger sister, along with my other siblings, would turn on the TV. We would move the chairs in the living room to the side, turn up the TV, and have a blast. Each person took turns as the lookout kid to watch out for our parents' return. When mother came down the street with her basket on her head, the lookout kid would shout, "Mommy is coming," as she rounded the corner. That would send us in a scramble as we turned off the TV and got all the furniture back in place. Then we went to our rooms and pretended as if we were reading a book or sweeping the house. Those were the good ole days.

Hearing certain songs reminds us of happy experiences with certain people in certain places. They bring back strong memories and the desire to go back to that place or to spend time with those people. I remembered much of the music that was played when I was in the early months and years of college, when I used to board off campus near the University of The West Indies (UWI), Mona. I remember the music that was played in the early days after meeting my first love, and we were invited to a birthday party where they played songs like "We are the world", "Lady in Red", and Celine Dion's "The Whispers in the Morning."

I remember many years ago when we could not afford to buy audio cassettes. We had a Walkman, which had a built-in recorder. So when we heard the music on our favorite station, we pressed the record button and taped the song. We stopped recording before the DJ's voice came on again. We would then make bootleg copies of it and share different combinations of songs with our friends. We were so happy when CD came around after the computer became more popular. Even though our family could not afford a computer, my friend had a computer and even a CD burner. He was the bootleg king of that time. He would burn his combination of songs of various genres in a way that there was no break in the songs. They flowed together is if a DJ were playing them.

The world have become obsessed with capturing live music for later playback. This can be seen in not only the evolution of musical instruments but also in the evolution of the recording devices we use to capture and transmit music. From the days of the phonogram, which was invented by Thomas Edison using a sheet of tin, to vinyl to the eight-track to magnetic cassette to CD to electronic media such as hard drives and USB drives to Bluetooth and the internet.

One of my favorite things to do is to sit and listen to music. I enjoy many genres, including country, reggae, hip-hop, R & B, soul, pop, and classical. There is something about music that sooths our souls. It is so amazing how they can take notes and beats and combine them into wonderful pieces of art called music, which can lift our moods from the lower planes to the synergistic master plane of bliss. It impacts lives, minds, and moods. Music is the soap that washes away the dust of everyday life from the soul, leaving us feeling fresh and clean in our spirits.

How do we know that a particular piece of music is out of tune? We seem to be born with an innate sense of what good music and musical arrangements are. Even without formal musical training, we can tell if a song is out of tune. Our minds just do not sync with it; we instinctlvely reject it.

Music is to the ears what a rainbow is to the eyes. Music is the oil that keeps the machines of our souls running smoothly. Music can unite people of different languages. Music intertwines with all aspects of our lives, so we spend billions of dollars on music and music-related activities and instruments. We have music in shopping centers and malls to create specific moods. We have music in our cars, in our homes, in our workplaces. Music is the universal medicine.

2.3 The Placebo: Belief Kills and Belief Cures

> You don't become what you want,
> you become what you believe.
>
> —Oprah Winfrey

People don't believe what they see; instead, they see what they believe. Imagination is the most powerful gift we have. Award-winning movie producer and actor Tyler Perry experienced a very traumatic childhood. He later said that his only escape was to imagine himself in a place of peace and joy to avoid the pain that he was experiencing. Later in life, he was able to build the life of peace and joy that he imagined.

It is said by Zeev Kolman in his book by the same title, that "Mind is the healer and mind is the killer." Your beliefs will become your biology. Centurions are future-oriented: As you live in the present, keep a futuristic perspective because learning takes place at all ages and stages of life. As a person thinks on a subconscious level, so he or she is.

Imagination

Everything already exists in the quantum or spirit realm. It is our faith and constant beliefs as we take action that cause us to realize the thing we imagined. What you imagine is imagining you.

To paraphrase what Abraham Maslow said, Never place anything in the imagination that you don't want to be actualized. Dr. Wayne Dyer said,

"If you advance confidently in the direction of your dreams, live the life you imagine, then you will meet with unexpected success."

Phantom Limbs and Mirror Therapy

No one has ever seen his or her own face. What a person sees is a reflection of his or her face in a mirror or other reflective item. Whenever a person loses a limb for any reason—be it a result of an accident, battlefield war, or surgical amputation because of an illness—there is sometimes a feeling or sensation that the missing limb is still there. Many such persons report that they sometimes feel an itching or pain where the limb used to be. When this occurs, it is called having a phantom itch or pain in a phantom limb. Pain is more likely if the person had a prolonged illness, like diabetes, before the limb was amputated. In many instances, the pain is severe and continuous to the point where they cannot sleep. This is a very real phenomenon that affects hundreds of people who have had an amputation. Many patients spend thousands on surgery, pain relievers, and therapy but with little or no success.

Much time and research have been invested in finding a cure for phantom pain. Medical science postulates that partial nerve fibers from the brain that would normally go to the now-removed limb are so convoluted, contorted, and splintered because of the abrupt or irregular termination that orphan nerves have been created. These orphan nerves fibers send distorted signals and pain sensations to the brain as the signals bounce back to the centers in the brain. This can be compared to an electrical circuit that is not properly terminated and shorted out as it sends sparks and blow the fuse in the main box.

One doctor was able to find a very simple and effective cure for some cases. He put the patient before a mirror so the patient could see a reflection of the intact limb. The sensation in the brain changed because there was now a complementary optical path to the signal. And they can now scratch or massage that part of their phantom limbs and find relief. This discovery has saved patients a lot of time, money, and pain.

Pain relief associated with mirror therapy may be due to the activation of mirror neurons in the hemisphere of the brain that is contralateral to the amputated limb. These neurons fire when a person either performs an action or observes another person performing an action. (Rossi S., F. Tecchio, P. Pasqualetti et al. "Somatosensory Processing during Movement Observation in Humans. *Clin Neurophysiol* 113:16–24.)

New England Journal Med 357:21, www.nejm.org, November 22, 2007.

The process of seeing has several components. The light that comes from an external object travels through the lenses of the eyes and lands on the film or retina at the back of the eye. The retina is connected via the optic nerves to the visionary cortex of the brain, where the image is interpreted. If there is a defect of any component along this path, it can affect our sight. For instance, if the lens, optic nerve, or visionary cortex is defective, vision can be impaired.

The interconnection of the visual and other neurons and how it plays into what we believe and how we interpret the physical world around us can be also seen in this other case. Tom, an older patient with relatively good eyesight can move around independently. But he has difficulty identifying Jane, his granddaughter. When she came to visit him in the nursing home and identified herself, Tom said, "I don't know you. My granddaughter doesn't look like you!"

However, when that same granddaughter went into another room and called him on the phone, he immediately recognized her voice and said, "Hello, Jane."

This aberration, called cortical blindness, is caused by damage to the visual cortex in the brain that affects the interpretation of images that come through the eyes. But in Tom's case, while his visual cortex may be damaged, the hearing path, including the auditory cortex, is intact, so he can identify his granddaughter based on her voice.

Blind Spots

There are many kinds of blind spots. There is a physical blind spot caused by damages of the optical components in the eyes or vision path that impair vision. There is a psychological blind spot of another kind that can impair our mental and emotional perspective. There is a vehicular blind spot related to driving where certain parts of the road may not be visible. One thing they all have in common is that they compromise our safety.

Based on our backgrounds and circumstances, we sometimes don't see things like other people see them. Sometimes we can be so prejudiced to the point that we are unaware that some words we use are insensitive and hurt others. Sometimes we can be willfully blind.

Cognitive or psychological blindness is when we are so caught up with and focused on certain things around us that we cannot see other things that are going on. The invisible guerrilla game proves that by getting someone distracted with certain things, they will miss other things happening in their environment.

I was driving on the highway one evening, and after checking my mirrors, I started to change lanes, thinking the lane next to me was clear. Before I was fully in the next lane, I suddenly heard a loud honk, so I pulled back in my lane so quickly that I almost lose control of the vehicle and hit the guardrail. In a few seconds, an angry lady with her kids in the car pulled next to me, and gestured at me. I felt so bad; I was so nervous. I could have hurt or killed the lady and her family, not because I was evil and wanted to, but because they were in my blind spot. I did not know that they were there.

When we travel on the highway, we see guardrails. What are they there for? Who needs them? Reckless drivers? Distracted drivers? Drunk drivers? Not necessarily. We all need guardrails. The vehicle in which we are traveling can malfunction and cause us to go over the cliff. Or someone else's vehicle can malfunction and cause us to hit a stone wall. So the guardrail acts as a cushion to slow the vehicle and prevent it and its occupants from sustaining major damages.

In the same way, we need guardrails for the subconscious, things that prevent us from going overboard and hurting ourselves. The subconscious is a very powerful engine. It does not question the instructions given; it just executes them. By having some guidelines and daily training, we can prevent ourselves from getting out of hand. By avoiding a slippery slope, we can prevent a skid, rather than having to try to control a skid in progress. For example, we may not want to hang out with certain people in the first place instead of hanging out with them and then try to mitigate the bad things you will get yourself into. There is an old proverb that says, "Keep your heart with all diligence for out of it flows the issues of life".

2.4 Meditation: Quiet the Mind

> The memory of God only comes to the quiet mind.
>
> – Jaime Fonte

The best time to meditate is when we first wake up and just before going to bed. These are the times when stress hormone levels are low since our minds are not focused on a million things. This is referred to as the delta state. The mind goes through several states as we wake up and fall asleep at nights. As we awake, we encounter the delta state, which is a very impressionable state. The next state is theta, which is still in the subconscious realm but just before we go in the conscious realm. Then the next state is alpha, which is the first state of consciousness, where we are neither calm nor aroused. The final state is beta, in which we are alert. A high beta represents a super-alert state, like being in a test.

Meditation Phase

To tap into the field of possibilities, we need to broaden our focus by shifting our attention from the immediate known environment and start sensing the vastness of the unknown. In meditation, we start with our attention on our bodies: the lower stomach to the heart to the throat to the head to above the head. Next, we sense the open space around our bodies and then the vastness of space filling the earth. We then move our attention to the planets and then beyond the planets and the cosmos. As we move our attention from the specific known to the vast unknown, our brains and bodies start to sync and become coherent. This can be seen in brain scans as the right and left hemispheres of our brains begin to connect and communicate. Additionally, the nervous system relaxes, and we begin to feel safe again.

As we linger in this state of being focused on the unknown, we begin to create new possibilities outside the familiar known or the predictable past because we are now creating from the field. Real creation can only take place as you tap into this field of possibilities. This source field transcends the physical 3-D world, and we must be on this frequency to tap into the field of possibilities. So moving our attention from the known to the unknown reduces our stress, allows us to connect with the energetic field, and for our minds to be flooded with new possibilities. This is similar to a tsunami, when the water moves from the shore due typically to a shift in the seabed and then later rushes back to shore in a vast wave, flooding the surrounding land and affecting new areas where no one previously thought possible for water to go.

When we envision our desires and goals while in a relaxed state, we automatically associate our goals with peace and joy. So we will be enthusiastic about planning and working on our goals. But on the other hand, when we try to envision our goals during a stressful time in the middle of the day, for example, we associate our goals with stress and anarchy. As a result, over time, we will not find it enticing to think about or go after our goals. Therefore, it is important to repeat aloud our written goals every day, just before we fall asleep. When we hear and see something repeatedly, it becomes familiar to us and less scary. When we have big goals, they can sometimes be scary. But as we become familiar with them, they don't seem so scary anymore. People are generally hesitant to approach things or people with which they are not familiar; we find it much easier to approach the familiar. Meditation is, by definition, to go over something repeatedly. The word "meditation" was derived from the chewing of cud, as an animal regurgitates the grass and repeatedly chews on it for several cycles.

Meditation is any activity that quiets or relaxes the mind and calms you enough to bring you peace. It could be listening to birds, watching the waves by the sea, or gardening. All thoughts carry an energy and a frequency that evoke the powerful subconscious, which is responsible for 95 percent of our achievements.

Collective consciousness for wholeness and health helps to reduce crimes in cities. It can also create abundance faster by removing emotional blockages. During our subconscious state, namely the delta state just before waking and just before falling asleep, we are more vulnerable to programming. This is when we create our lives. If we watch TV just before bed, with all the negative stuff like war, crimes, and corruption, it will seep deep down into our consciousnesses and program our minds. Don't let late-night TV program you. Job mentioned that the instruction we place in our minds is sealed in our thoughts when we sleep. The last five minutes before bed, don't think about the things that you don't want, are missing, who hurt you, or what's wrong. Use those last five minutes to go over things the way you want them to be, even if they are not that now.

Do the following steps twenty to thirty minutes each day if you are not busy. If you are busy, then do it for an hour.

Steps for Gratitude Meditation: Say, "Thank you," after Each Step,

- Close your eyes.
- Sit in a relaxed position.
- Relax the forehead and jaw that hold tension for overthinking.
- Relax the tension in the stomach, arms, and feet.
- Imagine the tension evaporating and melting away.
- Wiggle, shake your head and shoulders slowly.
- Envision bright lights coming into your eyes.
- Breathe deeply in and out. Imagine fresh breath coming through your body and lungs.
- Feel yourself releasing any resentment, anger, fear.
- Feel the lightness of who you are.
- Visualize your aura, your true expression connecting to others.

2.5 What Frequency Are You On?

> Your thoughts determine your frequency, and your feelings tell you immediately what frequency you are on.
>
> —Rhonda Byrne

Are our bodies controlled by chemistry or by energetic signals? Signals are transmitted in waves of frequency, which make them more powerful than particles. Use the mind to send signals of gratitude to the body, and watch how the number of immune cells increase. When we go back to past frustrations and feel victimized, notice how our minds send signals to depress our immune systems. For us to receive health and abundance, we must be on the frequency of love and gratitude. We cannot be on the frequency of hate and criticism.

There are many frequencies around us at any time, including those that carry radio waves on FM and AM bands, light waves, and Wi-Fi. There are even frequencies on the spectrum that humans cannot hear, but dog can hear. For example, those emitted by a dog whistle. There are transducers in our bodies that can pick up the vibrations of each of these frequencies and transmit them to the brain to be decoded as information. Sometimes frequencies from various devices around us may not be very good for us. Grounding can counteract the effects of cell phone and other radiation, so put your foot on the earth daily.

Energy Flows Where Attention Goes

The body has several centers of energy. Wherever there is a dense network of nerve tissues in the body, there is an energy center. The endocrine system maps the body's energy centers. There are basically seven centers which are like tornadoes which pull things in. The lower-energy centers consist of the gonads and the adrenal and pancreatic glands. The middle energy center is the heart. The higher-energy centers consist of the thyroid, penal, and pituitary glands. When we shift our focus from the lower centers to the higher centers, we increase the flow of energy within our bodies. As we release the energy from the lower-energy centers, energy travels up through the heart to the higher centers, where it best serves the body. Energies in the lower centers focus on survival needs, like procreation, nutrition, and fight-flight. But the energies of the higher centers are geared toward growth, development, and maintenance of the body.

Alignment with Assignment

Many years ago, when I was just a small boy, my father was in the process of doing an addition to our house. I understand the government of Jamaica had built these one-room "housing schemes" after the 1951 storm destroyed many houses in our area. By the time I was born, the third child, my parents had divided it into two rooms: one room for the bedroom and the other a dining room/living room. Close to the house, was an outside kitchen made of board and sheets of zinc with dirt floor. We used a wood fire before we could afford a kerosene stove. We had a wooden outhouse toward the back of the property and a place to bathe close by made of zinc. We needed to add rooms and inside bathrooms as the family was growing, and the kids were getting bigger.

When he showed me where the new walls were to be built, I was overwhelmed. I asked him how long it would take to build those walls. He told me, "Don't focus on the walls. Just focus on laying one brick at a time." And to my surprise, the walls were built before you knew it.

Many times we focus on the entire big project. And then we get discouraged and just give up. We needed to focus on one small, manageable unit of the process at a time. We basically need to ask ourselves, "What is the next small step I can take and not fail." As we do this repeatedly, we will come to a place of accomplishment. We must build by focusing on laying one brick on one wall at a time. Don't focus on the entire wall; that will discourage us. Also, we should not focus on building too many walls at once. We need to understand that life is a process.

My mom used to ask me, "Oral, did you do your homework assignment yet?"

"Yes, Mom," I would reply.

"Don't lie to me. I am going to ask Mrs. Grandison!"

It's the consistent accomplishing of the small task that gets us the big results. More recently, with the advent of social media, we see kids leaving high school thinking that they can build a brand overnight. But success means constantly working at your craft for a long time so we can get better at it. We come in alignment with our assignment or purpose when we take the time to do our due diligence, one small step at a time. This is how we come into full realization of our destiny.

Frequency of Abundance

Abundance is the flow or exchange of energy currency. When we have currency, we can exchange it for food, clothes, houses, and so on. When we get in the flow, our efforts are amplified. When a boat goes downstream, it uses less energy compared to when it is going upstream. What are some of the things that destroy one's abundance? One of the main things that destroys the ability to be abundant is the "enemy in me." That is, the enemy within, our self-saboteur. We think we are not smart enough or beautiful enough due to low self-esteem and negative self-perception.

It is important to note that most successful people did not start with smarts or education or sweat but with mentorship, support, and guidance from someone who was already successful in a particular area because we replicate the energy patterns of our peers to be socially acceptable and fit in. So when we connect with mentors who are already successful in the areas we desire to be successful in, it is much easier to flow in success. Every soldier needs an army, every player needs a team, and every bee needs a hive.

Parents program limitations during childhood, when the brain is in theta. So children automatically absorb the patterns, languages, and habits of our parents. Our brains are like sponges; they don't care what is in the environment, they just absorb it. Once we absorb the stuff in our brains, they create the set points and attitudes we have. As children, we don't question the validity of the stuff that is presented to us because we have no other frame of reference. We simply accept these habits so that we are acceptable to our parents. If we push back on our parents, we most likely will be reprimanded. From the child's perspective, he or she believes that to receive food and shelter, one needs to conform to parents' directives, whether the child likes it or not, whether they lead to abundance or not. How many times do we see children get spanked for not keeping within some so-called boundary or not doing something the way they were told by their parents, even if it is misguided?

Once these set points are created, they are nearly impossible to be removed after years of programming. Like a sponge that has absorbed ink and left to dry for years or weeks, you cannot get all the ink out of it. So this is how our set points or mindsets of lack and limitation are created. The result is that we talk ourselves out of good opportunities and overlook breakthroughs because of competing thoughts and undercurrents from our childhood programming. We then ultimately ignore the right people with wise counsel. Fear, distrust, doubt, hate, and criticism are on a frequency of lack.

These blockages are the enemies that destroy abundance and are subconsciously reenforced by society:

- Fear that you are abandoned by the unsafe world or God or fate.
- Doubt and belief that abundance is difficult to achieve.
- Distrust of God, seeing your job as the source when it is just a way to fulfill your passion and purpose, and to be rewarded.
- Belief that money or material possessions, such as a car, is the root of all evil. Money is the foundation of all good, and its usage for good or evil is an expression of who you are.
- Hatred and criticism of money and "those" rich people, not believing that you can become one of those rich persons.
- Belief that you don't need material things, only spiritual things, even though God works through currency.

Focused Meditation to Clear Blockage and Receive Overflow of Abundance

Connect to source energy, the safe masculine shepherd and caring motherly love, flowing from above to below. See the light of abundance coming into the following parts of the body:

- The head for clarity of thinking.
- The eyes for vision of possibilities.
- The ears to listen to good advice.
- The heart for gratitude.
- The hands for skill.
- The feet and hips to walk in the right doors of opportunities.
- The belly for conviction and passion.

Quantum physics say that when you observe something, it changes. When you look at something and have love and gratitude for it, you transform and bring it to you.

A hen sits on an egg and transforms it. Let us rest in the connection to the superconscious and be transformed from within. Let the blockages in our brains be dissolved. And let our brains become like sponges again to absorb abundance.

Connected to Source

Life consists of cycles: day and night, reaping and sowing. There is a water cycle and nitrogen cycle. When the cycle is broken, we experience distress as we become disconnected from source. The lack and disease we experience is often the manifestation of being disconnected from source, just like how a light bulb becomes dark when it is disconnected from the source of electricity. The light bulb is not defective. Someone may suggest that the light bulb be changed, but the that will not solve the problem. The tumor that you see is just a manifestation of being disconnected from the source of all goodness and abundance. Many times we hear about people who won the lottery and then become broke and sometimes bankrupt after a few years because the source of abundance is not in the cash, but in a mindset of abundance and how to invest money properly. Sometimes people have surgery for diabetes or undergo chemo for cancer, or treatment for a particular condition. After what appears to be initial success, the symptoms return after a while because they did not maintain a certain lifestyle and mindset of health, which is the root cause of health. In other words, they did not get on the frequency of healing and get connected to source.

2.6 As a Person Thinks

> As a man thinketh in his heart, so shall he be.
>
> —James Allen, "As a Man Thinketh"

Certain thoughts are associated with certain emotions, and certain emotions are connected to certain parts of the body. Therefore, whenever we are happy, we spontaneously smile or laugh without being asked to move the facial muscles to represent a smile or to make the sound of laughter. There is a physiological connection between certain emotions and certain parts of our bodies. Someone said, "Sad movies make me cry." Certain thoughts activate certain physical processes in the body. Just like certain thoughts can cause us to tear up, certain thoughts can make you sick, certain thoughts can make you sad, and certain thoughts can make you healthy.

Criticism, anger, resentment, and lack of satisfaction can trigger illnesses like cancer, and tumors. Many of the great moral teachers tells us that it is the things that comes out of our thinking that destroys us. Never talk about things you don't love. Rather, let us think about the things we love. We should never watch movies or listen to news that are full of negative elements. We become what we think and say continually. Change the way we think about ourselves, and we can change our lives because what we are not changing, we are choosing.

Reticular Articulating System—RAS

This part of your brain is like a strainer. It only lets in a small fraction of signals that are in our environment. It is impossible for the brain to process all the signals coming into it at any given time. This filter only lets in specific things that you are looking for. You can train it to look for certain thigs based on your thoughts and habits for it is a detective. For instance, if you are in a crowed, noisy mall and hear your name called, that information is let in. Essentially, it only lets your brain takes in things that are important to you, such as your name and other things that identify you, threats to health or safety, and procreating for survival needs, which is why you always notice an attractive person.

Don't let your brain let in negative stuff about yourself from you being too hard on yourself. Learn to high-five yourself, even if everything is not perfect. As a ritual, every morning after making your bed, hug and kiss yourself in the mirror, like how a three-year-old would go up to a mirror and embrace himself or herself. Challenge yourself to find something positive about yourself and in every situation. We will then find ourselves connecting the dots. This will put you in a completely different world psychologically.

When we don't love ourselves, we abuse ourselves with food, drugs, and alcohol. When we accomplish something, we must compliment ourselves. Sometimes we wait for our spouses or parents to tell us how lovely we look, and if they don't, we feel disappointed. Don't wait. We can praise ourselves.

As you focus on the positive, you will be energized. And if you focus on the negative, you will see, feel, think, and do devitalizing things. This sets the positive—or negative—intention for the day. We praise and pat each other on the back throughout our lives. We motivate others to be better and to play more skillfully. But why don't we motivate ourselves too. Don't see it as being selfish to put yourself in the middle. As we raise hands to high-five each other, we get in a posture to celebrate, so we receive and transfer energy that causes a dopamine bounce in our brains. Physical movement, such as patting on the back and embracing ourselves, causes new neural connections in the brain.

Think Yourself Worthy

What excuses do we give ourselves for feeling bad and going down familiar and negative paths? I'm too fat, tall, black, white, stupid, ugly? We need to stop the self-hatred and self-doubt and start declaring, "I am worthy of goodness. I deserve it." If you start to feel deserving, you will start to see evidence of your success. A recent study of various teams in a basketball league showed that those with the most high-fives and fist bumps did the best in the league. These activities are visceral actions that activate the dopamine centers and boosts the mood.

Start to act like the person who you want to become. Do not just think it; act it out as much as you can every moment that you get. Another helpful technique is to give yourself a positive new name if you dislike your name.

Taking steps every day is very important for daily momentum. It is not just the big win and then you slack off. You must get validation from yourself, not just from bosses or spouses, which, in many cases, does not come.

When your nervous system is on edge, it is difficult to function. A technique that I found useful during my recovery was putting my hands on my heart and communicating love, healing, and compassion to my heart every morning. The vagus nerve runs in the vicinity of the heart and controls the flight-or-fight response. As I practiced this, I felt calmer, more relaxed, and rested. Then my breath became freer. And yours will too. Experiments show that when a cat is eating in a cage and a growling dog is next door, the cat's stomach gets in a knot as it tries to digest its food. However, if the dog is not visible, even if it is still there, the cat's digestion is normal.

The greatest motivation in the world is loving, cheering, and encouraging, not criticizing, blaming, and shaming ourselves and others. Remember those coaches and teachers who screamed at you in anger? Even though you may have improved your performance, it left an unpleasant reminder in your consciousness. Anger is like nails that leave holes in a board even after the nails are withdrawn.

Humor and Kindness Heal Us

Notice that whenever a person hears a joke or something humorous, that person spontaneously breaks out into laughter and smiles without thinking about how to move his or her facial muscles to make the smile. In the same breath, if a person is angry, that person does not need to think about how to furrow the brow, for example. This is because our facial muscles and other parts of our bodies are primally wired to emotional centers with the ability to trigger certain psychological states. In short, our physiology is mapped to our psychology. So as we experience humor, we spontaneously cause certain energy centers of the body to be activated, and this improves our moods and cranks up our immune systems. Whenever I encounter situations where there is a lot of tension and sadness, I try to say something humorous. And suddenly, the mood is changed as everyone laughs.

Negative emotions and thoughts are connected to certain parts of our bodies. They can trigger sicknesses like cancer and cramps because emotions carry energy.

Whatever things are lovely, whatever things are of virtuous, these are the things that we should constantly think about. We should only think about things that we love, never about what we don't love. We should not listen to news that make us sad, and never watch movies that make us sad. We should not listen to or talk about the things that make us sad.

A man on a bus was sitting beside a lady whose bags were resting on him. But he decided not to say anything about it. Instead, he started to share a very encouraging story with her. The lady asked the man why he was not saying anything about the bags resting on him, even though they made him uncomfortable. He told her, "The ride is too short for me to spend time talking about something negative." He thought this brief encounter could be spent in a more positive way. He figured that if he started with the negative stuff, not only would he not have time for the positive stuff, but it would also probably leave a bad taste in her mouth, making her less likely to accept the positive encouragements. Life is too short for us to spend our time discussing negative things, listening to negative stuff, and thinking about inconsequential stuff. Let us focus our energy on the impactful stuff.

Studying the wrong answers to questions does not guarantee a pass on a test, especially if it is a fill-in-the blank test. Bank tellers are trained with genuine bills only, so as soon as a counterfeit bill comes, they can identify it because it feels and looks different, however slight the differences. Likewise, just by focusing on the positive things, we can quickly identify the negative elements in our lives and quickly eliminate them.

We need to use our time and resources wisely because they are limited for all of us. For instance, if you are given a thousand dollars to buy some stuff for your home, and you go to the store and find ugly, broken pieces of furniture and gadgets and purchase these until the money runs out, then when you get home, you will be out of money and time, and your house will be filled with junk. So we should not spend time and resources talking and thinking about things we don't love. Rather, talk and think about things we love.

Self-Unforgiveness Is the Ultimate Inside Job

Never speak evil of yourself or others, not even as a joke. Negative words are like spells cast over our lives. Words are energy, and the body does not know the difference between a joke and what is not. Even when we learn something negative about a person, it is our responsibility to cover and hide the evil of others—or at least don't say anything about it, especially when we are not asked or legally required to divulge that information. In that case, we can state the facts without passing judgment or evaluating a person's motives.

It is bad enough not to be able to forgive someone, but it is worse not to be able to forgive ourselves. Self-unforgiveness can keep us captive as we execute a destructive inside job of beating ourselves up year after year. Suppressed negative emotions are stored in the subconscious and can show up as knots in our stomachs or joints.

Suppressed negative emotions—such as anger, shame, guilt, disappointment, and resentment—cause us to seek and be attracted to negative situations and people to validate our negativity. So pent-up pressure of our negativity can be released like how one would release the built-up pressure in a pressure cooker. Have you ever seen a person explode and overreact to a situation? This is because we use projections to blame innocent others for our internal turmoil. They can act as triggers for our displaced emotions that thoughts and words create. The things that we hold on to, color our worldviews and perspectives. If you are sick, would you ask your neighbor to take the medication for you so you can feel better? Of course not! So don't expect your friends and family to change so you can feel better. You must deal with your own internal issues to feel better.

Despite our current conditions, we need to affirm the positive constantly. Let the weak say, "I am strong." As we get excited about our healing, it becomes easier for our bodies to be healed.

Affirmation: Remind Me of My Future

I understand and affirm that I am not my negative feelings. Negative feelings flow through me like a wind, and I observe them.

I will not hold on to them or suppress them. I will let them blow by.

Positive feelings are more a part of my true nature. They are the things that I will say yes to and give a thumbs-up to.

Negative feelings come from the stuff I naturally say no to and give the thumbs-down to.

I constantly affirm myself; I am positivity.

3

SPIRIT

How do we truly rest the spirit? How do we bring our spirits, these life-giving, animating parts of our beings that are regarded as the true self, this unchangeable part of us that transcends the physical, into balance to connect with source?

3.1 In-spirit-ation or Inspiration

> The soul always knows how to heal itself, the challenge
> is how to quiet the mind.
>
> —Wesley Speaking

When we act based on who we understand ourselves to be deep down, magic happens! Dig deep, find an aligned, congruent pure version of yourself, and take a stand based on that. When conflicted, one's inner sense of being diminishes, and chaos, destruction, and disruption happens.

Living to Be Me

The phenomenon of life after death—or more properly called "life after life"—has been reported by many individuals all over the world. These are situations where some individuals experienced trauma and may have lost physical consciousness or had a near-death experience. During this time, these persons report that their consciousnesses traveled and connected and communicated with friends and family from their past lives. One poster book example of this is Anita, who documented her experience in her book, *Dying to Be Me*. She had stage 4 cancer and was hospitalized in a coma. During her coma, she became aware of her dislike for herself, her inauthenticity, and fear was causing her cancer. So when she came back to physical consciousness, she started to live her life fearlessly and authentically. Within weeks, she was completely cured of her cancer. One of the major PBS networks carried her story as part of a documentary a few years ago.

As I mentioned earlier, when we are conflicted, one's inner sense of being diminishes, leading to chaos, unrest, destruction, and disruption. Have you ever noticed that it is difficult to do business successfully or to have a wholesome relationship with someone who is deeply conflicted? We can only truly feel we belong when we present our imperfect, authentic selves to the world in the present moment each day and not rushing into tomorrow to accomplish something. We should not be rushing into the future just to check the boxes. Instead, we must embrace ourselves for who we are today and be filled with gratitude for the air that we breathe and the space and form we occupy.

These medical phenomena of near death experiences are well documented in medical literature. Dr. Bruce Greyson is professor emeritus of psychiatry and neurobehavioral sciences at the UVA School of Medicine. He served on the medical school faculty at the Universities of Michigan, Connecticut, and Virginia. He was a cofounder and president of the International Association for Near-Death Studies and editor of the *Journal of Near-Death Studies*. His book *After* is the culmination of almost half a century of scientific research. He said, "The brain is a filter to let in only certain things that we need for our survival in this phase of our existence."

During the time of loss of physical consciousness, brain activity decreases, and mind consciousness rises. In these case studies, no psychedelic drugs were involved to change the person's states.

Greyson also mentioned that "Some of the effect of this near-death experience is that subjects became more compassionate and caring of others, more fearless and less attached to money, fame, materialism, as they come to understand that we are all from the one source."

The Impersonal Self

We are in this world but not of this world. The body is consciousness and energy. Both are formless and have no space-time dimension. The physical animation of the body that we see is a reflection, or hologram, of the real dynamics in the spirit realm, just like the sights and sounds we experience on a TV screen are based on a real-life scene in another part of the world, perhaps in another time frame. It would be foolish to think that we can correct the sound, for example, on the TV if the sound in the movie studio is out of whack. It would be foolish to think that we can change a sickness in our bodies if this sickness has a spiritual source. If we get into a place of quiet rest, we can connect to source and transform the holograms that are our bodies.

When the reproductive cells of our parents fused, there was a supreme intelligence that caused these cells to interact with each other that resulted in the cells' division to create different types of cells representing the different structures in our bodies. They multiplied again to create more of the same cells within a given structure until a perfect body was formed. All this happened in a peaceful, quiet, restful place independent of the mother's effort. If during this time the mother is in a place of unrest or chaos, the process could be disrupted, which could result in malformation or spontaneous abortion.

Muscle Testing

It is a verified phenomenon that when we are untruthful and dishonest, our physical bodies are weakened.

When I started to work with my naturopathic practitioners, I was introduced to muscle testing. For example, I would be given a bottle of vitamins or told to say something while stretching out my hand. My strength was determined by how much my hand could resist being pushed down. We proved that when I was insincere or inauthentic, I was weaker; my arm muscles were not able to resist being pushed down as effectively as when I was truthful.

Life can be very hustle and bustle as we run around in this rat race, being tempted to wheel and deal. We need to take time out to be in a place of rest and peace to strengthen ourselves.

Survival Mode

When we think something in our external environments can control or hurt us, or when we feel vulnerable to the external circumstances, whether a tiger or a virus, we go into survival mode. In this mode, we want to run or hide as the sympathetic system kicks in. Our immune systems are depressed as blood moves from the vital organs to outer extremities, and stress hormones flood the body. The ultimate desire of the soul is space and rest. This is one's eternal nature. Have you ever noticed how a child or an animal craves freedom? Living in this survival mode is not optimal. But we can be healed when we connect to the universal self and bring our entire beings into homeostasis. Sages of the ages who understood that they were the extensions of God, and who lived in a state of God-realization, were able to elevate their thoughts and bodies into the quantum realm and manifest healing spontaneously. And so can anyone of us if we come to the same God-realization.

3.2 Authenticity

> Time isn't precious at all, because it is an illusion. What you perceive as precious is not time but the one point that is out of time: the Now. That is precious indeed. The more you are focused on time—past and future—the more you miss the Now, the most precious thing there is.
>
> —Eckhart Tolle

In 1959 in Tennessee, a deeply racially segregated state, police were called on a nine-year-old, Afro-American boy who refused to take no for an answer when told he could not borrow a book from a library designated for whites only. Long story short, many years later, he graduated from one of the most prestigious educational institutions, MIT, with a PhD in astrophysics and later became a NASA astronaut. The school with the library was later renamed after him—the Ronald McNair Elementary School.

In 1985, he was the guest speaker at my high school graduation at Vere Technical, in Jamaica. The theme of his speech was, "Aim your gyro; correct as needed." This quote has inspired me over the decades. I have shared it with my kids, other family members, and friends. The word "gyro" references the gyroscope, a device used to measure or maintain orientation, angular velocity, or direction. This gyro has an internal momentum that doesn't change the direction in which it is pointing, regardless of how it is moved or turned. He used the gyro analogy to explain that as we move toward achieving our goals, deviations may occur that take us off course. However, if we focus on the goals based on where our internal guidance methods point us, we can make midcourse corrections and reach our desired destinations. In the *Wizard of Oz*, the cowardly lion, who was afraid of his tail, needed courage. Eventually he realized that the source of strength was not something external. The Tin Man was able to rediscover his heart after a wicked influence destroyed it. Don't be perturbed or changed by negative external circumstances created by others. In survival mode, we focus on external circumstances, but let us be steadfast, unmovable, always abounding in the work of advancing toward our destinations.

Who Are You?

At our very cores, we are consciousness or spirit; we are not just physical material beings. There is a part of the universal infinite consciousness in each of us. A consciousness called us into existence and continues to cause us to manifest our own unique identities. Take a red rose, for example. There is an awareness that causes it to open at a certain time and produce a certain color and fragrance. This red rose is not trying to be yellow rose. The same essence that directed it to open directs it to close, and there is nothing any of us can do to stop that process.

Humans have organs and features that grow unsolicited in unique ways. This growth and path are from that divine within. Get in a quiet place, listen to the inner voice of consciousness and follow the path it is taking you down. Don't worry about outcome, opinions, or opportunities. It is not about how much money you can make or who will love you. Self-actualized individuals do what they do because they know deep down that they are supposed to do this special thing and fulfill their destinies.

How Do You Identify Yourself?

If you identify yourself in terms of the changeable material world, that is not your real identity. Your real identity is not changeable.

When I was a child, I used to dig the earth in the backyard to find premium clay to make toy cars. On some occasions, my siblings would join me, and we would make clay pots, cups, and saucers for our toy house. We baked these toys in the open sun on metal, such as paint pan covers. If we found any paint left from our father's work, we painted the toys. If the toys got broken, we would be so sad because we would say that the toy no longer existed, even though the same clay and paints still existed. So if our identities are tied to material stuff that changes, then we would cease to exist when our body changed. However, we do continue to exist beyond our bodies.

Together we constitute the collective consciousness that transcends time and the material world. This consciousness finds its expression in love, laughter, light, and life.

We will enter rest when we learn to accept ourselves and to dance with the gifts the universe bestowed on us. Let's look at three birds with very distinct characteristics: the eagle, the peacock, and the hummingbird. The eagle has a wingspan of up to nine feet and rarely flap its wings. It soars in the air above the clouds, make loves in the air, and has powerful eyesight and night vision. But it is not as colorful as, say, the peacock. On the other hand, the peacock has a beautiful, expansive tail and illustrious feathers. But it cannot soar above the clouds. The hummingbird has small wings that flap thirty times a second and a long beak that it uses to extract nectar from flowers. But it cannot spread its tail like the peacock. Each of these birds have their unique characteristics and each of these birds are happy in themselves. They are not going around trying to be the other. For us to be happy and fulfilled, we need to stop tormenting ourselves by looking at and comparing ourselves with other people's "feathers." We need to focus on accomplishing what we were placed in the world to do. Stop measuring your feathers against those who come along next to you. Stop being overly introspective, and you will be brought in the company of greatness.

Authentic Relationship

Due to my immaturity, the relationship with my partner went belly-up just before the 9/11 attack on the WTC because I did not understand my unique and authentic responsibility to create my own happiness.

Even when we are in a relationship, we must embrace our uniqueness. We came from different backgrounds and have different perspectives on life. We cannot be overly dependent on each other to make us happy. Instead, we each whip up and create our own happiness and bring it to our relationships. That is, we don't come with our cups begging for handouts of happiness. We come with our cups overflowing with happiness to give to each other to drink from. Not only is it unfair, but it is also destructive to place the responsibility of your happiness on someone else's shoulder. You need to take responsibility for your happiness. You cannot blame and shame another for not making you happy.

We have so many misguided perceptions about love and relationships. We often enter relationships with the wrong intentions, ulterior motives, or hidden agendas to fulfill pressing needs. But true love is about serving and giving value to the other so that your partner becomes all he or she was meant to be. It is not forcing or demanding them to become who we want them to be to suit our ego needs. It is letting the other blossom into the most authentic expression of himself or herself. If we approach a relationship with the mindset of, "If you fulfill my needs, I will love you," the relationship becomes contractual and feels transactional. The greatest pleasure in this world is not food or travel or money or sex. It is giving service to others in a loving and sincere manner.

A great way to find out who a person is, is to ask him or her:

- What TV character reminds you the most of yourself and why?
- Which cartoon character do you most identify with?
- What drives you? Not what you want to be later in life, but what motivates you now?
- Who do you admire as a role model?
- What have you accomplished in the last year?
- What do you hope to accomplish in the next year?

3.3 Faith Conquers Fear

> Fear is corrupted faith.
>
> —Denzel Washington

Faith is the substance of things hoped for. Believe that you can get well and succeed, and it will likely happen. Imagination helps to make the unfamiliar familiar. The brain relishes the familiar and more readily executes the things you are convinced of. If you present something unfamiliar to someone, the individual is more likely to be fearful of it and reject it. If you are walking on the street and a stranger comes up into your face, you may be fearful and step back. But it if is someone you know, you will embrace the person.

In the same breath, if you present your dreams and goals to yourself and they are not familiar, you are more likely to pull back from them and reject them by procrastinating. Therefore, it is important that you spend time every day in meditation, envisioning yourself in the role of your dream so that you can become familiar with it. This meditation should be done just as you wake up, before the mind and body start to experience the stress of the day. It should be repeated at night, when you are about to go to bed and are calm. As mentioned earlier in this book, the time just before you fall asleep and just before you awake is also called the "delta doorway" because the mind in the delta state can transform the conceptual into the physical. If you try to meditate during the stressful time of the day, you will automatically associate your dreams and goals with stress and anxiety. If you associate your dreams with stress, you will feel very stressed whenever you think about your dreams and will be less likely to go after them.

Life Is a Self-Fulfilling Prophesy

Your thoughts and imagination can reduce or increase your immune response. Fear is the house of cards built by your despair. Every decision we make is made from either fear or love. Are we eating what we believe to be the right kind of food because we are afraid of getting sick? Or are we eating those foods because we love them and are passionate about them? Are we married to someone because we are afraid of being poor and lonely? Or are we truly in love with the person and the idea of being in a relationship?

Love, not fear, keeps you safe. Live your life fearlessly and authentically, and whatever is truly yours will come to you. Even when you are ill, you should still think about health because everything exists simultaneously in the quantum field.

A narrow focus is very stressful and requires a lot of energy. But when we relax, focus expands. When an animal like a deer is under attack by a tiger, it needs to have a very narrow and specific focus on the attacker to determine its speed and position. The deer also needs to focus on an escape route and hiding place. It will not be paying attention to all the other wonderful things happening in the environment. This is a stressful time for the deer.

For survival purposes, we have evolved to have and associate a very narrow focus with stress. We can expand our awareness and take our focus off one specific thing to be conscious of other realities. We can see a bigger picture, as if there was a floodlight pointing at everything at once.

Infinite possibilities exist on the spectrum of life at any given time. Among them are possibilities for abundance, lack, health, sickness, sadness, happiness, and so on, as well as many variations in between. Some people are experiencing one or more of these possibilities. Which of these possibilities are you experiencing now? Even if you have experienced one or more of these possibilities at various times. But the key question is what factor determines which possibilities you experience or where you end up at any given time? It is your faith. Faith is like a currency. For example, when you have currency, you can exchange hunger and lack for food; when you have currency, you can exchange homelessness for a house.

Faith is the energetic currency that can converge a specific possibility that exists in the field of possibilities to a specific possibility in the real world.

After being bedridden with severe respiratory illness and eczema, I had the faith to believe that there was a possibility of being healed, which I could experience. I held on to that belief in my gratitude meditation each day until I experienced the convergence.

In honor of Eczema Awareness Month of October, actress Tia Mowry shared her story with *People* in hope of raising awareness for those who might be suffering from eczema that had not been properly diagnosed: "Eczema is definitely a chronic condition that's very prominent within the African American community but unfortunately, there's a huge percentage of people suffering with eczema and it actually goes underdiagnosed. And that happens to be a part of my story. I'm definitely a part of that percentage."

Faith Moves in Waves

Waves have specific properties, like amplitude and frequency. The frequency of a wave determines its signal or message. This is why different radio stations carry different messages. The wave's amplitude determines its power. This is why a powerful hurricane can produce huge waves on the seashore that come on land and destroy buildings. If the amplitude of the wave is small, the effect is small. But if the amplitude of the wave is large, the effect or damage is large. The level of one's emotional excitement does determine the power of his or her faith. So when we combine some specific information (frequency) of what we need with the level of our excitement (amplitude), we can experience resonance, and our entire beings are moved into wholeness as sickness and lack are dispelled. The level of faith is determined by the level of emotional excitement; that is, specific actions of joy and gratitude. Without the proper level of excitement, we will not experience that shift.

Two waves can either be constructive or destructive to each other. Whenever two waves have the same frequency and are going in the same direction, the result is a bigger wave; this is called constructive interference. Conversely, if they are moving in the opposite direction, the result is a smaller wave or no wave at all. Even though faith moves in waves, we should be careful not to generate counteracting waves that could destroy or cancel our positive forward moving waves. That is, faith. One of the things that destroys faith is doubt. Doubt is shown in the form of a lack of emotional joy and gratitude about what is coming to us to the point that we don't take action toward our goals. If we truly believe that something good is coming our way, why wouldn't we be excited? When we truly believe that we are about to receive something or have received something valuable and important, then we will be exuberant and elated. We would be filled with gratitude! We can cancel our dreams with negative emotions. The joy of the supernatural is our strength.

Posture and Position

We often don't realize how powerful we are and what we can accomplish until our backs are against the wall, and we are put in a position in which we need to get out of a dangerous situation. When I was a teenager at VTHS, I was only able to jump about three feet over the high jump bar. However, one day I was on my way from school and took a backroad shortcut home through what appeared to be an empty wasteland. Lo and behold, as I stepped across the path and was in the middle of the field,

I saw a bulldog bounding toward me. I knew I needed to run. I quickly surveyed the area with the hope of finding the shortest path out. Luckily, this was a fence just a few yards away. So with the dog now at my heels, I breathlessly sprinted toward this five-foot barbed-wired fence, wondering how I would get through it since there was no room to crawl under it. In any case, I probably did not have enough time to do that. I decided to literally take a leap of faith and made a big jump in an attempt to go over the fence. That was my only option. Time slowed down as it seemed like I was in the air for an extended period. I believed I can fly! I made a crash landing on the ground on the other side of the fence. I was sure I ripped my skin against the fence, but to my surprise, I was scratch-free. The dog was not able to clear the fence, so it stood there, barking at me. I teased him by kicking at him through the fence before I left. When we position ourselves to do something, like surmounting difficult obstacles, we will most likely succeed even though it may seem impossible at first.

The mind is very powerful. It is said that "As a man thinks, so is he." When we are about to do something, we need to get our minds in a posture for it, and the body will follow. For example, when I am traveling with the kids, I usually ask them to use the bathroom before we get in the car, so we don't have to stop on the way. Most of the time, they will say that they don't want to, but a few minutes after we start out, one of them will cry out, "Bathroom break!"

I then yell out, "Didn't I just ask you if you wanted to use the restroom a few minutes ago?"

"Yes, Dad. But I did not want to use it then."

Now, before we leave home, I have learned to mandate that they go in the restroom and get into position, even if they don't feel like it. And guess what? Most of the time they will use it, and we don't have to stop on our short trips. So, if we want something in life, we need to get into that mental posture, and we will be surprised how doors will start to open for us. We will begin to feel and see things that we did not feel or see before. Many skillful ballplayers seem to develop an instinct for the game and have learned to be in the right position, in the right posture, at the right time to play the ball for a winning game, be it soccer, tennis, football, or basketball.

If you want to be happy and abundant, a good place to begin is to put yourself in that position mentally and, as much as you can, physically. That may mean you put yourself around happy people. It may mean you should wear clothes that make you feel abundant. It may mean you should stand and walk like someone who is joyful and abundant and talk like a champion. It is said that physiology follows psychology. In other words, one's physical state of being follows his or her mental frame of mind.

Research shows that whenever we stand in a superhero posture instead of slouching, our immune responses increase. Therefore, many toy companies, movie producers, and cartoon makers use the superhero posture, with head high and chest out. There are many examples of people in the world who were healed from issues by getting into that mental position through belief.

Phobias and How to Overcome Them

While some fears are reasonable and justifiable, many are not. There are times when we truly need to be afraid of certain things, for example, for our protection. Some fears developed from the existential need for protection and survival, while others developed from negative childhood experiences with an object or situation. Excessive irrational fears are called phobias. Individuals affected by the phobias will go to great length, over and beyond to avoid the situations that trigger their irrational fears. Such phobias include xenophobia, which is the fear of strangers, and even PTSD.

What fears were we born with, if any? It is believed that the only fear we were born with is the fear of falling. A stressful event causes us to subconsciously create a permanent recording of the circumstances surrounding it. This snapshot typically includes the time, place, and characteristics of the person or thing that was involved. Later, anything that remotely resembles what originally scared us brings back the memories and emotions of hurt, loss, and disappointment. So essentially, whenever we experience fear, we are taking the energy of the present and investing it in the past, since all fears are born out of past experiences or something similar to a past experience.

Irrational fears cause us to do irrational things. They may even cause us to hurt ourselves or others unjustly and unjustifiably.

Perfect love drives out fear. Sometimes we can even be fearful of stepping into something like a promotion because we are not familiar the role, even though we are capable. However, as we spend time in meditation, we see ourselves in the role and become comfortable and familiar with our destinies and hence, less fearful. We can then step into things and get intimate with things that originally scared us.

As we digest the bad news from the media, we become conditioned to negativity. It is said that by the time a child in the developed world reaches adulthood, he or she will have seen thousands of images of crimes on TV, radio, and other media programs that, in fact, "program" the mind into this habit of fear. While we should be aware of the events going on in our world, we don't need to immerse ourselves in certain levels of details about remote events that have little or no effect on our lives. We should not spend an inordinate amount of time and effort digesting negative information, especially just before we go to bed and immediately on waking in the mornings. These are the time we are most susceptible to absorbing information and being programmed.

Fear in the body shows up as elevated blood pressure and levels of cortisol and other poisonous substances that harm the body over the long run. The body cannot distinguish between a real fear and one that is imagined. Phobias take away precious mental and emotion energy as we divert energy that could go into planning and moving forward on our goals. Instead of living in fear, let us invest our attention on gratitude for the wonderful things we have in the present.

An experiment was done in which cells were placed in two petri dishes. Nutrients were added to one and poison to the other. The cell with the poison stopped growing and went into protective mode in an attempt to preserve itself. Fear is the protection mode where we go into lockdown, but growth is the open mode where we expand. We see that we cannot be in fear and growth at the same time.

3.4 Vision Transcends the Past

> Are you going to be defined by a vision of the future or
> are you going to live by the memories of the past?
>
> —Joe Dispenza

Vision is seeing things that we would like to happen in our lives before they happen. The placebo effect is essentially an act of faith that is manifested in the body. The negative effect of negative thoughts on the human body are very real, and the converse is true. A man used humor to cure his illness, and it was discovered that morphine is released in the brain when we are happy. We should not talk about negative feelings or give them much attention, or they will stick to us and become our friends.

Whenever something negative—like, "You are stupid," or, "You cannot do that," or, "You are too dumb," or, "you are too ugly"—is said to you once, do you know that you need to hear something opposite at least twenty times for you to believe otherwise? Yes, a child needs to hear that he or she is smart at least twenty times to even start believing that he or she is not stupid, after being told the opposite.

Negative things we hear are buried deep in our subconscious minds. It takes repetition over time to displace them with positive stuff. This is because as we hear things over and over, we start to visualize ourselves in these roles. We start to envision ourselves doing the things we thought we could not do. This can be enhanced through meditation, quieting the mind to rehearsing the positive stuff. Seeds develop in the dark under the earth; eggs develop in the dark when the mother hen sits on them for days in a quiet place. It is difficult to do things you don't first envision yourself doing. To meditate is to become familiar with, so as we meditate, we move away from the negative past and the depressing predictable future. We become more familiar with our authentic selves in the present. Yesterday is gone, and tomorrow is not here. We only have the present to enjoy our presence.

Smash that Mirror

Some mirrors may make you appear shorter or taller than you really are. That is, they give you a distorted view of yourself. The images we develop about ourselves are borne out of subconscious programming. It is great to know we can smash those mirrors that give us distorted views of ourselves and go back to one that truly reflects our authentic selves. We have been receiving that programming from the time were born. In fact, even before we were born, when we were in utero. According to Dr. Bruce Lipton, a spiritual teacher and epigeneticist, "During the first couple years of life a baby is in the delta brain wave state. This is a state that is very susceptible to programming." That is why it is so easy for kids to learn a second language while it takes an adult a much longer time and with great difficulty.

By the time we are seven years old, we are already programmed for life into the person we have become, unless we undergo some radical psychological transformation. Much of the programming at this stage is from our archetypes: parents, siblings, and teachers. The subconscious programming are habits we develop that pretty much seal our destinies. The subconscious mind is like a car engine, and the conscious mind is like the driver. Wherever the driver directs the car to go, it will go with great speed and power—no questions asked—whether it is in a ditch or into another car on the road.

However, it is important to understand that genetics do not determine one's final destiny. We don't have to be the products of genetic determinism. The signals we provide to our biology will be the final determinant of our destinies.

The Blame Game

We tend to direct our attention away from our own weaknesses instead of focusing on improving ourselves. Why do we criticize others? In part, because we don't want to take responsibility for our lives. Everyone needs to take responsibility for their actions and their consequences. By pointing fingers at others, we justify and validate our failed states, thus giving us an opportunity to say, "Well, look how terrible that person is, so, I am not so bad."

Additionally, we criticize others because pointing fingers is *easier* than doing the work to improve our conditions. It's easier than planning or starting a business or going back to school or going to the gym. Criticism allows us to take the easy way out. People who criticize others are always looking for ways to release the social pressure of not achieving when they should be further in life.

Furthermore, we criticize another because of self-hate as we seek to avoid the embarrassment of being alone as an underachiever.

We must release criticism because it reflects a desire to control others and not to change ourselves. If you point a finger at another for your condition, you are giving your power to someone else. You will not be able to change until that person releases you. But he or she may never release you, and you will be stuck for life. All of us have people who hate us and wish that the earth would open and swallow us. But we cannot focus on the haters. We need to get over it and declare affirmatively, "It is up to me, and no one can stop me from walking into my destiny!"

Whenever you are tempted to blame or criticize someone, always ask yourself, "Is there something that I can do right now, right here, with what I do have to make my situation better?" Then focus on that, and get to work on it.

'Dis-ease' with Destiny

We are sometimes uncomfortable with new levels of destiny or where we are going. For example, a person may have the ability to become a manager or sit in a boardroom, but because he or she is uncomfortable, the individual will walk away from opportunities to develop a career. This disease with destiny can cause us to talk ourselves out of good opportunities and to overlook breakthroughs because of competing cross-thoughts and undercurrents. Or we ignore people with wise counsel. Bishop T. D. Jakes, an entrepreneur, motivational speaker and movie producer, called this, 'dis-ease' with destiny.

Bishop T.D. Jakes further states, "This is why it is important to take time out to write the vision" that is flowing from our most intense desires. For it to be most effective, we need to read the vision aloud just before going to sleep and as soon as we wake up. As mentioned throughout the book, this delta doorway is when the vision can truly be assimilated into our subconscious minds. As we become familiar with where we are going, we are most likely to step into our destinies.

Write It, Read It, Run It

One of the great things about writing our vision is that it gives us clarity and perspective on our goals. Studies show that when we proactively write our goals, we are 70 percent more likely to execute them. It is not enough to use our heads as journals or filing cabinets for our visions. Also, if we write or draw them with pen and paper, we are more likely to accomplish them. Furthermore, if we make a movie about our goals, using for instance an app on a smart phone, we are even more likely to accomplish it. On several occasions I wrote my vision and marveled to see the speed and accuracy with which it came to pass. Many years ago, I wrote that I wanted to work in tech and teach. Within a year after, I was offered several positions as a tech professor at several colleges in my state. I have also seen this materialized in my living space, transportation, organizations, and relationship.

It is important to put pen to paper and document our deepest desires of where we want to go and what we would like to do if money, time, or any other resource were not obstacles. This creates a big picture of the direction we want our lives to go in. Our vision statement is not a statement of our needs, problems, obstacles, or past pain. Rather, it is a forward-looking statement covering the important aspects of our lives, including our spiritual lives, emotional lives, intellectual lives, and our family lives. It also includes financial, recreational, and physical desires, as well as how we want to contribute to humanity. We can also even write the vision about how many likes and views we would like to get on social media.

Whenever we go to a restaurant, we place our orders with the waiter or server and don't run into the kitchen every minute to check to see if the chef is cooking our food. So we should place our orders with the universal chef and believe they are coming to us and we get into the position of gratitude. We must make our orders big, bold, and grand. Our visions must be articulated very clearly and in as much details as possible, without worrying about the details of how it will be accomplished. I guarantee that in time, we will see them come to pass, as we discover creative steps to execute them.

Our thoughts are like rippled waves created when a stone is cast into a pond. We don't know the extent of these waves of thought or where they will eventually go. Thoughts are like a spark placed in a forest; it can set aflame thousands of acres. Our visions are like seeds that can be picked up by the wind or a bird and transported to another part of the world, where it can get lodged into the soil and grow to be a massive tree that produces more seeds and other trees. It is said that a flutter of a butterfly wing can create a storm on the other side of the world after a certain time. This means that the small thoughts and actions we take now can have a tremendous effect later in life in other places of the world. The intentions we put out into the world will come back to us, usually in a different form. Take, for example, Colin Powell, a great American statesman, soldier, and politician. His parents came from Jamaica, but he was born in Harlem, New York and went to public school and city college. He made history as the first African American to head the joint chief of staff of the US Armed Forces, as well as the first black man to be secretary of state. He said that we should be consistent and follow our dreams, and we will achieve our goals.

The mind sends out thought waves that cannot be seem or registered on conventional equipment. There are many sights and sounds that are not perceptible on the current electromagnetic spectrum. There are many frequencies that cannot be perceived by our physical senses. For instance, X-rays cannot be seen with the naked eyes, but they can be picked up on film sensitive to the imagery. Radio waves, though invisible to the human eyes, can be picked up by the transducer in a radio. In the same breath, thoughts can be sent out by our minds and picked up by others. We thereby experience serendipitous encounters to fulfill our visions. For example, a young man saw a high-end car that he loved and took a picture of himself in the car, which he then posted on his social media pages. A few years later, he came to know the owner of the car dealership, who took him to his house and gave him an unbelievable offer on a car of the same make and model as the one he placed on his social media page.

Thoughts create waves that can be registered subconsciously as changes in our brain waves and heart rhythms on an EKG. That is why we have lie-detector testing machines with varying levels of reliability. Our inner talk and thoughts create our outer world experiences. A wise teacher said that our words proceed from our conscious and subconscious thoughts and eventually determine our lives.

3.5 Ascendence

> The oak sleeps in the acorn. The bird waits in the egg, and in the highest vision of the soul, a waking angel stirs. Dreams are the seedlings of reality.
>
> —Napoleon Hill

Love and compassion produce spiritual impulses to the soul that cause vibrations and give direction so that you transcend the weight and baggage that weigh you down, thus allowing you to soar like an eagle. You must creatively remove things that don't serve you anymore. Are you living under the weight of illusion of someone's opinion and thoughts about you? Whenever we have a thought, it produces tiny impulses of electricity that travel to different parts of our bodies through the nervous system. These impulses can heal or sicken us. Our thoughts are like sound waves in a cave that go out from our lips and bounce back to us in the form of echoes. Our thoughts go out into the world and come back to us as positive or negative experiences based on whether our thoughts are negative or positive.

Cocreators of the Universe

There is divinity within each of us. The Creator created this beautiful world and placed us in it to be cocreators with him. He did not create tables and chairs, but he created the trees and gave us the knowledge of how to create tables and chairs from the trees. We have been given the power to be cocreators.

While airplanes and cell phones may be relatively new to us in the sense that they were been created relatively recently in the span of existence, if you had told someone a few centuries ago that you were going to use a little device, about two inches by four inches, and talk to someone on the other side of the world, that person would think you were crazy or an angel or a god of some sorts. But today, that is common practice. You pick up your cell phone, and in a few seconds, you are talking to and can see someone on the other side of the world. Likewise, a few years ago, if you told someone you were going to do a day trip to the other side of the world, you would again have been told it was impossible. But today, we regularly fly from one continent to another in under a day. We even have sent spacecraft to the moon and Mars, both millions of miles from earth.

For years, fire was used for light and cooking. But then, with the inventions of new and more efficient ways to create light and to cook, fire fell by the wayside. However, when we rediscovered fire and harnessed it in new and creative ways, we were able to create the internal combustion engine that transformed the steam engine and is used in cars and airplanes today. Of late, we have been able to trap the sun or solar energy and harness it in even more creative ways to propel rockets to the outer space.

But the materials from which they are created are not new. These materials have been around for millenniums, but we are just gaining the knowledge of how to transform those materials into new devices and gadgets. And there are so many wonderful things that are yet to be invented or created from the existing material placed on this earth by our Creator.

There is divinity within each of us. We have the power to take an apple and by eating it, transform it into human tissues and cells. As we become more intelligent, we become more powerful as we leverage our inventions. Centuries ago, you would need an army to destroy a city. Now, with the press of a button, one person can destroy the whole earth. Therefore, it is important that we stay conscious and connected to the source of all good so that we can preserve this creation we were given and not pollute it.

When the world is polluted because of unrest, it become useless or even dangerous. When we overcultivate the land and do not give it enough rest cycles, the land gets depleted of nutrients and does not produce foods with the level of nutrients our bodies need. And when this happens, death and disease set in as our planet gets tossed in chaos and clutter. But we can begin to create order by first decluttering our minds, bodies, and spirits. Start to create order with the small things, like making our beds when we get up each day and keeping our surroundings clean and in order. We can then take this to our places of work, worship, and pleasure. One of my friends mentioned to me that he decluttered his room, and his indigestion went away after many years. And shortly after, he landed a new job. Self-actualized people have a higher consciousness and are detached from the outcomes of their efforts.

The laws of the material world don't apply to the person of higher consciousness who is God-realized or living in the quantum realm. They see only love for those who hurt them. Undiscriminating virtue and service are the only virtues that will allow you to reach the angelic realm, where you receive guidance and direction from your better angels. These angels cannot be bought or sought. Only they can seek you.

The self-actualized person calls those things that are not as though they were. If you are sick, see yourself as if already healed, and watch how the universe offers an experience you thought you could only imagine. Don't wait for your healing to feel healed; don't wait on your marriage to feel loved; don't wait on your wealth to feel abundant. You are creating your experiences through your feelings. Enriched people have a burning desire to do the things they are passionate about.

How May I Serve?

There is an omnipotent spiritual force at our fingertips. It contains the solutions to our problems and gives us self-awareness for tapping the healing energy within all of us. When we allow the ego to get out of the way, and give our bodies, our time, and our treasures in the service and advancement of the greater good—like healing other people's sorrows and salving wounds—miracles will happen for us.

Wayne Dyer got healing in both his knees, which were scheduled for replacement surgery, after he helped a paraplegic man by carrying him on his back. He previously wore braces, and on one occasion, was carried off the tennis court after his knees buckled. He had recently been diagnosed with severe cartilage erosion and damage in his knee to the point that bone was rubbing on bone. However, he received an instantaneous healing as he offered to carry this 170-pound man on his back up a flight of stairs. As he was healed and felt the strength in his knees, he was able to run with a man on his back up the stairs at the monument of St. Francis of Assisi. So the question we should be asking is not, "How do I become rich," but, "How may I serve?" Many of us are waiting on God to heal us or to give us abundance. But since we are waiting on God, then we are truly "waiters," and waiters serve. Therefore, while we wait on God, let us serve each other.

The External Self and the Death of the Old

Many people are afraid to move on or die because we think that is a terrible thing. Whenever a person thinks of moving on, he or she often becomes scared that he or she will lose significance and go into nonexistence. This is because of the misinformation they received, sometimes from well-meaning people. There is an eternal self that existed before we came into our present bodies. It will exist after we leave these bodies. When we are released from the limitations of the body, we will move at the speed of light and fly on wings of angels.

Take a little girl of, say, three years old, who is being advised by an adult. She is being told that she will have a much larger body than the one she has now, so her nice shoes that used to fit her won't fit her anymore. She may become sad because she is worried about losing her shoes. She is told that she will leave her mom and go into a far country to live with someone she doesn't even know now, and she gets scared. While all these future changes are factual, they may be scary for a little girl. But we don't need to be scared because our transformations will be out of this world as we evolve with time.

While it is important to know when a wave is coming and be able to ride it, it is also important to know when a wave is dying, so you can jump off and not to go down with the wave.

Opportunities Are Created from Adversities

Life is a matter of perspectives. The many problems we encounter every day can either destroy us or advance us. Research shows that as we encounter our Goliaths, one of two things can happen. First, we can be so scared that we shrink away from our problems. Or we can be so riled up that we are motivated to conquer the situation we face.

Shortly after the attacks of 9/11, there was a heavy feeling of depression caused by the knowledge that our world was under terrorist attack. As a result, the Peace Corps gathered in New York City for several days to send out energy of love, peace, and tranquility. This helped reduce the feeling of depression for many.

In the past, whenever this group went to a part of the world troubled by natural or human-made disasters and sent out positivity, there would be a scientifically measurable drop in crime, accidents, and violence. The more individuals who participate in this and the longer and more intensely that they send out this energy for good, the more pronounced were the results of the change. The subconscious mind is a source of invisible energy and can transform our bodies as well as our minds, and ultimately, the world. Like any source of energy, the more units of energy and the more intense the energy, the greater will be its effect of creating changes.

3.6 The Dance of Bliss

> Activate the neurochemistry of bliss in your own brain using specific meditation practices that have scientifically proven to produce dopamine, serotonin, and other blissful chemicals.
>
> —Vishen Mind Valley

Have you ever wished that you could escape to a place solitude and quietness to experience bliss? Well, you don't have to escape from the reality of friends and family and work and stay in a monastery for twenty years with your legs crossed to have that experience constantly. We chase happiness by getting into relationships and buying things because bliss and happiness are the goals. Even though we experience daily setbacks that can change our moods, through neuroplasticity we can permanently create changes in our brains to be in a state of bliss every morning we wake up.

Your brain can be trained to rapidly come into that state of blissfulness. In that state, there is better right brain to left brain coherence and heart coherence. The brain's waves take on a distinct gamma frequency. Dr. Dorson Church did several case studies on these transcendent brain states.

Your day-to-day baseline for happiness and productivity changes for the better, and this is reflected in your social and emotional lives as states become traits. Our local minds now merge with the infinite mind. When you get in the flow, you readily create new things, you feel more at peace and connected, and you more quickly and efficiently solve complicated problems at work, in relationships, or at school.

When we rest, several neurochemicals are released that correspond to these states. These include dopamine, oxytocin, and serotonin. These states persist for several days after rest and meditation.

Restorative healing culminates with recreation. This is the dance that remakes the entire person into a new you. We experience joy and happiness beyond our wildest imaginations. Everyone seeks to be joyful and fulfilled, though in different ways. Some of us seek it by going to a temple, some of us seek it in a bar, while others may try to find it in shopping for more things.

Happiness is superficial because it depends on what happens to you. But joy emanates from deep down and is more permanent. External material things don't necessarily make you joyful. If you don't have intrinsic joy, what does it matter if you increase the square footage of your home? Or drive a faster car? When the body, mind, and spirit are fully rested and aligned, we can experience true bliss. When the body is rested, we experience bliss as a pain-free agile body. When the mind is rested, we experience bliss as peace and tranquility. When the spirit is rested, we experience bliss as a connection to the superconscious self.

The essence of bliss is not to want to be somewhere else but to be present in the moment and enjoy the quietness where we are right now by connecting with things in the here and now. It is to tame the ego, be detached from the results, think small while we advance confidently in the direction of our passions.

Enthusiasm

What is the role of our emotions in determining who or what we become? Do our emotions affect the things we attract? Our emotions connect us to the field of infinite possibilities through waves of enthusiasm. The word "enthusiasm" comes from the Greek word "in" and "Theos"—God. Thus enthusiasm, means to be engulfed and infused with Theos and is a heavenly state of being. When we are infused with elevated emotions of love, joy, peace, and gratitude, we become lightning rods for favor and grace. These emotions send ripples of energy through our various organs to create healing. This is the dance of bliss. Whenever we are depressed and frustrated, our homeostasis states are disrupted, and the hormones that create sickness increase. However, whenever we are joyful, all the healing hormones run throughout our bodies. Our thoughts can make us sick, and our thoughts can make us whole.

What are you passionate about? Enthusiasm relates to passion. When you are passionate about something, you can do that thing for extended periods without getting board or tired. You will think about what or who you are passionate about for many hours of the day for many weeks, sometimes years. For example, if you are passionate about cooking, the preparation aspect of thinking about what and how to cook is just as important as cooking the meal itself.

Passion is what the impersonal voice within is calling you to do. This will be different for each person, but it will always be exciting to see a person do something with passion or to speak about his or her passion. What you are passionate about will animate your life and spirit, giving meaning and purpose to your existence.

Why are some people so negative in everything that they do and speak? I believe people can only give what they have inside them. How can we give a dozen oranges if we don't have a dozen oranges? We can only give a dozen oranges if we have them. So whenever people are always negative and hateful, it is only because that is what they have inside them. When people have love inside them, they can freely give love and kindness and compassion.

Whenever we squeeze an orange, only orange juice can come out; we can never get pineapple juice from an orange. Whenever we are squeezed, only what is inside us will be exuded. Sometimes we think that it is our circumstances, and the thing squeezing us is responsible for what is coming out of us—the juice. If we want to change the negativity that exudes from us, we need to change what's inside us.

Sacred Teaching

A good man out of the good treasure of the heart brings forth good things: and an evil man out of the evil treasure brings forth evil things. TD Jakes once said, "For out of the heart proceed evil thoughts like criticism, hate, and deceit." It should be our deep-down desire each step of our journeys to spend time in quiet meditation, communicating with our hearts before we jump out of the bed each morning, and ask for a clean heart and renewal of a right spirit within us.

Emotions

Emotions, more than intellect, govern our actions. Emotions are stronger than intellect. This can be seen in situations where a person knows intellectually he or she needs to stop doing something harmful, like smoking, but just cannot do so because of how it makes him or her feel, at least temporarily. The way to overcome this is by piling on massive positive emotional associations for the things we like and want to do. For example, if you want to stop overeating late at night, you may have to constantly associate overeating with sickness.

One's IQ, or intelligence quotient describes how smart we are in respect to a person's ability to learn and master the sciences, mathematics, law, medicine, and so on. However, what is equally important, or more important in some cases, is or EQ, or emotional quotient. This describes how smart we are with respect to the ability to read the emotional elements of a situation and control our emotions so that they do not get the better of us. This ability allows us to be engaged in better verbal and nonverbal communication. EQ is needed to properly and effectively network with team members and customers across a wide spectrum of personalities. It allows us to deal with difficulties in a cordial way and not burst into temper tantrums, like an infant, when things do not go our way.

Gratitude

Gratitude is the big boomerang. Whatever we give thanks for, we receive in return. It is sowing or giving out to the universe, and whatever we sow, we will reap multiplied.

Many times our slowly becomes a suddenly. There is a biblical story of a man, Lazarus, who was sick for many days, and his sister requested the healer to come and heal him. However, the healer was delayed, and so the man died. But when the healer arrived, he raised him from the dead. So, Lazarus got a miracle instead of a healing. Whenever we experience such a life-changing miracle, we should not keep it to ourselves. Instead, we must go tell it on the mountain. By sharing the good news of resurrection and transformation, someone could think, *If that person received a miracle, then I can receive a miracle too.* Lazarus's sister, Mary, advocated for him. It is good to know that someone, a friend or relative, can advocate for us and help us get to the point of wholeness when we are challenged. Do you know the plan God has for you? If Mary knew that the plan was to raise her brother from the dead, she would not have been weeping.

Sometimes we may even need to be pulled up by the arm. Another biblical story tells of a man who was lame sitting at the gate of a temple, begging for handouts as people passed by. When Peter and John saw him, they authorized him to rise and walk. They grabbed him by the hand and lifted him. From that time, he gained strength in his feet and ran all around and celebrated. It is customary that whenever you receive something, you give thanks. Don't wait for your breakthrough to start giving thanks. Don't wait for the oil of wealth and prosperity to start flowing before giving thanks. Don't wait for your family or your body to get sick before you remember, appreciate, and give thanks for them. Raise your level of your gratitude to have the oil of favor and joy flow down upon you. Gratitude brings you into wholeness. By opening channels on the frequency of healing, gratitude brings you to the concert to hear the symphony of joy.

Some folks say that when they see the miracle, they will believe it. However, when we believe it, we will see it. Though the situation looks bleak, we should still trust the universe that it is for our good, and good will ultimately come out of every situation. Though the fig tree shall not blossom, though there may not be any present good that we can stake our claim on, we can be happy because we know that good will eventually come out of any situation.

Gratitude replaces negativity with optimism and positivity. If you feel grateful to be alive, you won't be angry about slow traffic. Gratitude gives perspective on handling the bad things. There are some games that I have seen on the internet called "distraction" games. The setting of the rules for you to focus on certain things causes you to miss other important things in the game. This is because the RAS filters important external signals to the brain, so let us filter in the positive things of life and be grateful for them.

When we express gratitude verbally, we participate in the phenomenon of voice activation. Voice activation is used in several of today's technologies. Through affirmations, our thoughts go out and come back to us as reflections in the form of experiences, just like an echo. A farmer plants the seed in the ground, and the earth pushes it out in the form of a plant. Cast your seed into the ground. It will come back to you.

Gratitude must be expressed either written or spoken. It is the "Open Sesame" of life. At the gate to the cave where treasure was stored, Ali Baba overheard one of the thieves say, "Open Sesame!" The stone that blocked the cave rolled to the side, giving access to the treasure. The word also refers to the sesame seed that pops open when mature. Gratitude is the voice-activated password that grants access. It is the ticket that will get us into the concert, it is the coupon that will get us the discount, and the passport that will get us entry into the land of our dreams. Enter with the key of thanksgiving into the gates of heavenly abundance. If you can't give thanks for the small things, you will not give thanks for the big things.

I heard the story of a man whose daughter became sick and could not go to college. Before her illness, he was unable to see and be grateful for the many little blessings in his life. Little things like just having a cooked meal, having a house to live in, and waking up to see his family in the house. Before her illness, he was easily upset about any little thing that went wrong, like traffic, snow, and a broken faucet. After her illness, he realized nothing else was important or worthy to be angry about. He was so grateful to be alive and to have a daughter, even though all her friends had gone to college and were telling her about the wonderful time they were having. He must forget anger and focus on being kind and grateful to the people around him now. This was a powerful lesson in gratitude for him.

Gratitude is the ultimate state of receiving. Whenever we receive something, we give thanks. When we give thanks for something that we have received in our spirits, we must also give thanks even though we don't see the physical manifestation. As we give thanks, we put our bodies and emotions in a state of receivership and health. This is the difference between poverty

RESTORATIVE HEALING BEGINS WITH REST

and gratitude thinking and talking. So let us continue to affirm that wealth comes in faster than it goes out and believe this is not vanity thinking. When we indulge in cutthroat, disrespect and stealing, we are saying we cannot be abundant except by dishonesty. Criticisms of wealth don't endear it to you or make you feel comfortable embracing it.

Rest for a reset. Even though my mental, emotional, physical, spiritual, financial, and relationship health were destroyed, I was able to be restored by resting my body, mind and spirit. Rest to be restored to the ultimate state of bliss. Restoration begins with rest and ends with recreation.

Lightning Source UK Ltd.
Milton Keynes UK
UKHW011236140622
404414UK00001B/161